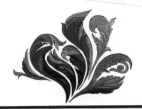

Hatred, Emptiness, and Hope

TRANSFERENCE-FOCUSED PSYCHOTHERAPY IN PERSONALITY DISORDERS

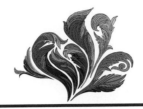

Hatred, Emptiness, and Hope

TRANSFERENCE-FOCUSED PSYCHOTHERAPY IN PERSONALITY DISORDERS

By

Otto F. Kernberg, M.D.

Director, Personality Disorders Institute,
New York Presbyterian Hospital, Westchester Division
Professor of Psychiatry, Weill Medical College of Cornell University
Training and Supervising Analyst, Columbia University Center for
Psychoanalytic Training and Research

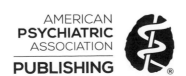

AMERICAN
PSYCHIATRIC
ASSOCIATION
PUBLISHING

Copyright © 2023 American Psychiatric Association Publishing
ALL RIGHTS RESERVED
First Edition

Manufactured in the United States of America on acid-free paper
26   25   24   23   22   5   4   3   2   1

American Psychiatric Association Publishing
800 Maine Avenue SW, Suite 900
Washington, DC 20024-2812
www.appi.org

Library of Congress Cataloging-in-Publication Data
Names: Kernberg, Otto F., 1928- author. | American Psychiatric Association
      Publishing, issuing body.
Title: Hatred, emptiness, and hope : transference-focused psychotherapy in personality disorders/ by Otto F. Kernberg.
Description: First edition. | Washington, DC : American Psychiatric Association
      Publishing, [2023] | Includes bibliographical references and index.
Identifiers: LCCN 2022013016 (print) | LCCN 2022013017 (ebook) | ISBN
      9781615374618 (paperback) | ISBN 9781615374625 (ebook)
Subjects: MESH: Personality Disorders—therapy | Psychotherapy—methods |
      Transference, Psychology | Object Attachment
Classification: LCC RC554 (print) | LCC RC554 (ebook) | NLM WM 190 |
      DDC 616.85/81—dc23/eng/20220412
LC record available at https://lccn.loc.gov/2022013016
LC ebook record available at https://lccn.loc.gov/2022013017

British Library Cataloguing in Publication Data
A CIP record is available from the British Library.

To Kay, once again, with love and gratitude

CONTENTS

Introduction ix
Acknowledgments xiii

PART I
Major Theoretical Statements

1 Object Relations Theory and
Transference Analysis 3

2 Some Implications of New Developments
in Neurobiology for Psychoanalytic
Object Relations Theory 15

PART II
Technique

3 Extensions of Psychoanalytic Technique
*The Mutual Influences of Standard Psychoanalysis
and Transference-Focused Psychotherapy* 35

4 Therapeutic Implications of Transference
Structures in Various Personality Pathologies 61

5 Affective Dominance, Dyadic Relationship,
and Mentalization 95

6 Reflections on Supervision. 113

PART III
Specific Psychopathologies

7 Psychodynamics and Treatment of Schizoid
Personality Disorders. 133

8 Psychotic Personality Structure 147

9 Narcissistic Pathology of Love Relations 165

PART IV
Application of Object Relations Theory

10 Psychoanalytic Approaches to Inpatient
Treatment of Personality Disorders
A Neglected Dimension. 191

11 Malignant Narcissism and Large Group
Regression. 213

12 Challenges for the Future of Psychoanalysis 233

Index. 251

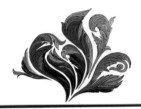

Introduction

The present volume continues my investigation of the psychopathology and treatment of severe personality disorders. It focuses on the analysis of particular clinical features of personality pathologies and describes contemporary psychoanalytic object relations theory as a general theoretical frame of treatment that allows us to conceptualize both normal personality functioning and the very nature of personality disorders. This volume also includes my recent contributions to understanding the relationship between neurobiological dispositions and their interaction with psychodynamic developments, again, both in normality and psychopathology. Finally, this volume explores the application of object relations theory to group processes, love relations, and therapists' training.

Part I of the book includes major theoretical statements. Chapter 1, "Object Relations Theory and Transference Analysis," presents a brief, updated summary of contemporary object relations theory and its direct relevance to transference analysis, the fundamental therapeutic approach of transference-focused psychotherapy (TFP). This chapter summarizes the theoretical approach that informs the new psychotherapeutic developments in the treatment of severe personality disorders that are described throughout the entire volume. Chapter 2, "Some Implications of New Developments in Neurobiology for Psychoanalytic Object Relations Theory" summarizes developments in neurobiology regarding the conceptualization of affect systems and their role as the motivational basis for establishing internalized dyadic self- and object-relations structures. This chapter shows how the underlying limbic and cortical brain structures and functions contribute to embedding the fundamental concepts of self and of significant others. It proposes that the formation of such dyadic structures is an essential task of higher levels of psychic functioning.

Part II, on technique, updates empirical studies of the Personality Disorders Institute at Weill Cornell Medical College, expanding the applications of TFP, exploring its relationship to standard psychoanalytic technique, and outlining a general comprehensive theory of technique that applies to both psychoanalysis and its derived psychotherapies. Chapter 3, "Extensions of Psychoanalytic Technique: The Mutual Influences of Standard Psychoanalysis and Transference-Focused Psychotherapy" presents an updated view of TFP in comparison with standard psychoanalytic technique that differentiates more sharply these two technical approaches and discusses the problems in training therapists efficiently in both modalities. Chapter 4, "Therapeutic Implications of Transference Structures in Various Personality Pathologies," presents an overview of transference developments in different modalities of severe personality disorders and the modifications in technical approaches to transference analysis related to these structural differences. It is a highly specialized description of TFP in action. Chapter 5, "Affective Dominance, Dyadic Relationship, and Mentalization," focuses on two basic premises from which the therapist enters every therapeutic session—that is, the alertness to affective dominance and the diagnosis of the predominant dyadic object relationship linked to it. By illustrating this approach with clinical cases, the chapter also points to similarities and differences between TFP and mentalization-based therapy (MBT), an alternative psychodynamic approach to severe personality disorders. Chapter 6, "Reflections on Supervision," describes my personal experience as well as general controversial issues regarding the supervision of psychoanalytic and derivative treatments. In the process, the chapter details our collective experience of training and supervising clinicians in TFP over many years at the Personality Disorders Institute.

Part III, on specific psychopathologies, deals with particular disorders within the broad field of severe personality disorders. Chapter 7, "Psychodynamics and Treatment of Schizoid Personality Disorders," presents our experience with these complex disorders. Schizoid structure has received less attention in recent times than other types of severe personality disorders, particularly borderline and narcissistic personality disorders. This chapter presents a diagnostic update and summarizes the specific contributions of the TFP approach to the treatment of schizoid personality. Chapter 8, "Psychotic Personality Structure," explores the differences between borderline personality organization and psychotic personality organization. It describes the development of psychotic features as a potential transitory regression in patients with borderline personality organization, as well as a reflection of a psychotic structure that only emerges during treatment. It proposes corresponding differences in technique for transitory psychotic developments arising in sessions, for transference psychosis, and for the emergence of major psychotic illness during the course of TFP. The chapter also analyzes the nature and shifts in reality testing in the context of transference analysis. Chapter 9, "Narcissistic Pathology of Love Relations," deals with the specific pathology of narcissistic personalities, the great difficulties of these patients in establishing and maintaining a love relation in depth, and the general study of sexuality and the capacity to love as part of the diagnostic evaluation of all patients with severe personality disorders. It also considers the influences of the therapist's own emotional maturity in the assessment of this aspect of psychopathology.

Part IV deals with the application of object relations theory to inpatient hospital treatment, to group regression and political leadership, and to psychoanalytic education. Chapter 10, "Psychoanalytic Approaches to Inpatient Treatment of Personality Disorders: A Neglected Dimension," examines the inpatient treatment of patients with personality disorders, a neglected therapeutic approach in the United States. Although pioneered predominantly in the United States, inpatient treatment has been developed in new ways in recent European experiences, with relatively extended hospital treatment of severe personality disorders. This chapter summarizes both the North American and recent European experiences with an important therapeutic instrument that, mostly for financial reasons, has been underutilized in the United States. It offers important technical tools that are relevant for the repetitive brief hospitalizations of regressed borderline patients that have replaced selective long-term inpatient treatment. This approach may be the basis for the development of optimal treatment of very regressed stages of illness in the future. Chapter 11, "Malignant Narcissism and Large Group Regression," applies psychoanalytic object relations theory and the developing knowledge of the social functioning of some personality disorders to the study of the mutual influences of severe leadership pathology in organizational and political structures and the psychological conditions that underpin large group regression. Political circumstances that foster such large group regression in social subgroups and leadership with malignant narcissistic features tend to reinforce each other, with potentially damaging and dangerous consequences to the social community. This chapter is a contribution to the clarification of these potentially threatening and damaging social developments. Chapter 12, "Challenges for the Future of Psychoanalysis," applies the psychoanalytical approach that underlies this volume to the analysis of particular conditions of psychoanalysis today as a profession, an educational enterprise, and a social organization within the mental health sciences. This chapter and the book end with recommendations for innovations that may strengthen the role of psychoanalysis as a profession, a treatment approach, and a social organization. It proposes solutions to organizational problems, particularly stressing the urgent need for development of empirical research, psychoanalytic psychotherapies, and radical renovation in its educational structure.

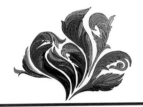

Acknowledgments

I have been privileged by my personal relationships with distinguished psychoanalysts and psychiatrists in the past whose influence continues to inspire my work at present, although they all have left this world— Drs. Betty Joseph, Andre Green, Joseph Sandler, Anne-Marie Sandler, Ignacio Matte-Blanco, Edith Jacobson, and Martin Bergmann. I am profoundly grateful to them, and they continue to be active in my mind.

Colleagues and friends in the United States who continue to inspire and encourage me include Dr. Harold Blum, Dr. Robert Michels, and Dr. Robert Tyson. Dr. Michels' critical review of my work, always available when needed, has been essential. In Germany, I have had creative and stimulating interactions over many years with Dr. Peter Buchheim, who has been a crucial support and influential leader in communicating my work and the work of our Institute within the German language countries, and with Drs. Susanne Hörz, Mathias Lohmer, Philipp Martius, Rainer Krause, Almuth Sellschopp, Agnes Scheider-Heine, and Gerhard Roth. Dr. Roth, in particular, is a distinguished neuroscientist who has stimulated my thinking about the neurobiological determinants of the self-structure. Dr. Peter Zagermann has focused on institutional complications in teaching psychoanalysis and psychoanalytic psychotherapy, and Dr. Martin Engelberg on the administrative and political dynamics of social organizations. Dr. Manfred Lütz inspired me to explore the spiritual aspects of dyadic relations and their connection to religious convictions. Dr. Rainer Krause alerted me to the subtle and complex communicative aspects of affect expression. The European community of transference-focused psychotherapists includes distinguished psychoanalysts and professors of psychiatry, including Dr. Stephan Doering, leader of this community in Europe; Drs. Melitta Fischer-Kern, Peter Schuster, Anna Buchheim, and George Brownstone in Austria; and the late Dr. Gerhard Dammann in Switzerland. The recent loss of Dr. Dammann, a pioneer in the contemporary approach to the inpatient treatment of personality disorders and an expert on schizoid pathology, has been a painful personal experience. Other members of the psychoanalytic community who have stimulated my interest and influenced my work include Drs. Anna Maria Nicoló and Paolo Migone in Italy, Drs. Claudio Eizrik and Elias da Rocha Barros in Brazil, Dr. Sara Zac de Filc in Argentina, and Drs. Ivan Arango and César Guerrero in Mexico.

The members of our European community of TFP experts who have influenced particularly my empirical research work include Drs. Massimo Ammaniti and Chiara De Panfilis in Italy and Drs. Miguel Angel González-Torres, Alfons Icart, and Luis Valenciano in Spain. My work has been significantly shaped by the work of researchers and professors in the mental health field such as Drs. Nancy McWilliams, Vamik Volkan, Salman Akhtar, Michael Garrett, and Peter Fonagy. Dr. Mark Solms has deeply influenced me with his incorporation of Jaak Panksepp's work on the neurobiology of affects as directly related to the psychoanalytic theory of drives. Panksepp's detailed description of affect systems and their basic motivational role in human psychology, together with Dr. Gerhard Roth's influence, have deeply inspired me to explore the boundaries between intrapsychic structure and neurobiological determinants.

By far, the greatest influencers on my work, providing ongoing challenges and stimulation as well as profound encouragement, have been the members of the Personality Disorders Institute at Cornell, and my deepest gratitude goes to them. First of all, Dr. John Clarkin, co-director of the Institute, has fundamentally directed our empirical research, has constantly challenged me to explore the behavioral aspects of intrapsychic functioning, and has stimulated related research throughout our international TFP community. Dr. Eve Caligor carried out important enrichments of our technical approach to the entire spectrum of personality disorders; Dr. Frank Yeomans has effectively directed our national and international educational activities; and Dr. Diana Diamond specialized in the study of attachment and narcissism and their importance in the field of psychoanalytic object relations theory. Our research collaboration with Drs. Mark Lenzenweger, Michael Posner, David Silbersweig, and Kenneth Levy in the United States has been essential. Our specialized adolescent personality disorders group, which includes Dr. Alan Weiner in New York, Drs. Lina Normandin and Karin Ensink in

Canada, and Drs. Marion Braun, Werner Köpp, Maya Krischer, and Irmgard Kreft in Germany, are vigorously developing our approach to personality disorders in adolescence and expanding it to the study of personality disorders in children. Drs. Monica Carsky, Richard Hersch, Eric Fertuck, Catherine Haran, Michael Stone, Barry Stern, Nicole Cain, and Jill Delaney, the senior members of the clinical and research team at the Personality Disorders Institute, are carrying out important clinical and research contributions and jointly have been an ongoing source of new ideas and efforts that have helped me develop my own work. I am particularly grateful to Ms. Jill Delaney for her personal help in the careful and detailed editing of this book, for her teaching of psychodynamic psychotherapy, and for her inspired organizational capacity with directing all our major conference work.

The technical support of my work has been carried out efficiently by Mrs. Janie Blumenthal, who diligently typed and organized the chapters of this book. I also wish to express my heartfelt gratitude to my personal secretary and longstanding former administrative secretary at the Personality Disorders Institute, Ms. Louise Taitt, who over the years has provided me with caring protection of my time, shielding me from many administrative and bureaucratic temptations and guarding my time for creative work.

All of this would not have been possible without the strong, trusting, stimulating, and protective support of the chairpersons of the Department of Psychiatry of Weill Cornell Medical College, particularly, throughout the years, Drs. Robert Michels, Jack Barchas, and Francis Lee. Dr. Lee, who is presently a professor and the chairman of the Department of Psychiatry, has strongly encouraged our work and is watching over our future, and I feel very grateful to him.

I also wish to express my profound gratitude to the late Mr. Alvin Dworman and to the Dworman Family Fund, who have generously contributed to the finances of our research enterprise, and to Dr. and Mrs. Michael Tusiani for their confidence and generous support of the Borderline Personality Disorder Resource Center, our educational support center for patients with severe personality disorders, their families, and the therapists who treat them.

Last, but not least, I want to thank my wife, Dr. Catherine Haran, who, in her double function as a senior clinician and researcher at the Personality Disorders Institute and as a loving provider of unfailing emotional support under all conditions of professional institutional weather, has helped me to produce this book. This work is dedicated to her as an expression of my profound love and gratitude. The experience of our life together has profoundly influenced the section on love included herein.

PART I

Major Theoretical Statements

CHAPTER 1

Object Relations Theory and Transference Analysis

Psychoanalytic Object Relations Theory

What follows is an overview of the essential theory and technique of transference-focused psychotherapy (TFP), a modified psychoanalytic treatment geared to the treatment of individuals with personality disorders, particularly severe disorders. TFP is a psychodynamic psychotherapy derived from psychoanalytic principles and techniques and represents an extension of the psychoanalytic model to cover the entire range of severity of personality disorders. It is based on a contemporary formulation of psychoanalytic psychotherapy, updated in the light of both empirical research and scientific developments in boundary fields close to the psychodynamic endeavor, particularly affective neuroscience and the psychology of couples and small groups (Yeomans et al. 2015).

Classical psychoanalytic theory proposed that the etiology of personality disorder symptoms and a broad spectrum of symptomatic neuroses—including depressive reactions, anxiety syndromes, sexual difficulties, particular inhibitions, and severe disturbances in interpersonal relations—were all related to unconscious intrapsychic conflicts derived from pathogenic developments during infancy and childhood. These unconscious intrapsychic conflicts essentially develop between libido and aggression—that is, the fundamental drives described by Freud as the basic human motivational systems—on the one hand and the infantile reality-imposed defenses against them, the mechanisms of defense centering on repression and related defensive operations, on the other. The discovery of primitive defensive operations centering on splitting and related defense mechanisms predating the dominance of repression and the division of mind into a defensive "ego" as opposed to a repressed "id," permitted the clarification of the earliest structure of the mind. These structures centered on dissociated idealized and persecutory internalized object relations, reflecting respectively libido and aggression. Thus, the notion of libido and aggression (or the death instinct) as basic sources of intrapsychic conflict, and the enormous influence of unconscious intrapsychic factors in maintaining and expressing them as neurotic symptoms and pathological character traits, mark the essence of classical psychoanalytic theory.

In light of today's knowledge and understanding, this basic formulation must be modified. Neurobiological research has demonstrated the key functions of primary, inborn, genetically determined, and constitutionally given affect systems as primary motivational forces, perhaps best classified in models of positive and negative affect systems. Positive affect systems include attachment, eroticism, and play bonding, or a general affiliative urge directed toward other members of the same species. These are positive, pleasurable affect systems that motivate the organism to develop relations with significant others to gratify the basic psychological need for positive emotional connections. They combine longings for dependency, erotic intimacy, and affiliative enjoyment and jointly constitute what Freud described as *libido*. The negative affective systems of fight-flight and separation-panic jointly constitute what Freud described as the *aggressive drive* or *death drive* and represent the entire spectrum of negative emotional dispositions. In addition, an exploratory or searching affective system reflects a general interest in actively exploring the environment that may reinforce the corresponding systems upon gratification of any positive or threatening activation of any negative affective systems. From a broad biological perspective, affect systems permit the survival of the individual and the species because they motivate the individual to seek nourishment, protection, social cooperation, and security and ensure the reproduction of the species while equipping individuals to fight or escape from harmful stimuli or environmental dangers. Affect systems thus constitute homeostatic mechanisms that operate beyond the need for intra-organismic control, such as maintenance of temperature, blood pressure, and elimination functions, by expanding homeostatic control over psychological functions that equip and require human beings to be in intimate touch and to negotiate their needs with other human beings.

This modification of classical motivational psychoanalytic theory from the original dual drive theory into one based on the neurobiology of affect systems culminates, however, in the eventual integration within individuals of the positive and negative affect systems in the context of their interactions with other human beings. Clinically, the unconscious struggles involving love and aggression as supraordinate integration of positive and negative affects reflect the basic nature of unconscious intrapsychic conflict that must be discovered, understood, and resolved in the course of psychotherapeutic treatment (Kernberg 2018).

Another significant change in the classical theory of unconscious intrapsychic conflict is the discovery of multiple functions of unconscious mental processes that constitute a dominant etiological factor for much psychopathology. These processes include the cognitive integration of sensory perception, of procedural memory to maintain homeostatic functions such as learning skills, and of the specific unconscious declarative memory processes that reflect the unconscious conflicts mentioned earlier—in other words, the dynamic unconscious motivating the development of psychological symptoms and personality disorders. We now assume the origin of the dynamic unconscious resides in primary conscious affective experiences in the interaction between infant and mother—that is, in the impact of conscious affect activation. Because the infant hippocampus is immature prior to the second year of life, this central neurobiological structure involved in affective, long-range declarative memory storage is not yet available. Therefore, these early affective experiences leave learned skills and behavior patterns but no subjective experiential evidence. This is the cause of infantile amnesia. Only after the second year of life can the split between positive and negative affective experiences remain consciously available. This occurs under structural intrapsychic conditions that may express intrapsychic conflicts at a conscious but dissociated level via defensive operations based upon splitting. Idealized and persecutory internalized object relations are represented in subjective split experiences. Only in the third year of life and with the achievement of identity integration will repressive mechanisms dominate. Intrapsychic conflicts will then become the dynamic unconscious ("the id") in a concrete sense. Thus, the dynamic unconscious, in its advanced form of truly unconscious, repressed pathogenic conflicts, only covers the advanced intrapsychic structures of psychopathology related to these conflictual dynamics. In short, the concept of the dynamic unconscious has evolved into complex stages of psychological development that each have different ways of organizing intrapsychic conflicts and defenses in general (Kernberg 2021).

Psychoanalytic object relations theory proposes that the activation of conflictual affect systems related to unresolved dynamics from the past is always expressed as a particular experience of the individual's "self" in relation with a significant "other" under the impact of a dominant affect. In other words, the activation of affects always involves the activation of a subjective interpersonal experience, positive or negative, and the expression of this experience in the relation with a significant other or object. A specific experience of the self is always connected with a specific experience of the object and thus constitutes a fundamental psychological entity that, through declarative affective memory, remains a core feature of the subjective nature of psychological functioning. Units of positive and negative affects and their corresponding self and object representations are the "building blocks" of the mind. Their integration leads to the gradual achievement of an integrated self, interacting with significant others and, in turn, reflecting integrated positive and negative views of those others. Psychoanalytic object relations theory, in short, proposes that the internalization of significant relationships between the self and others under the impact of peak affect states is the fundamental dyadic infrastructure of the mind.

Consolidation and gradual integration of these dyadic units into more complex, supraordinate structures lead to the development of the tripartite structure of ego, superego, and the dynamic unconscious (the id) and are reflected in the specific organization of the functions centered in the self (ego), the repressed sector of a conflictual and repressed dynamic unconscious (id), and the buildup of an integrated system of internalized ethical regulations (superego). This understanding transforms the traditional psychoanalytic tripartite model into a sequence of stages of internalizing component dyadic, and subsequent triadic, object relations structures. These basic internalized dyads are conceived as originally framed in peak affect states, both positive and negative, determining, respectively, "all good" and "all bad" idealized and persecutive mental structures that, under normal circumstances, are eventually integrated into the tripartite model.

The concept of an integrated self includes the autobiographical awareness of self, together with imagination and planning (the time dimension of self experience) in the context of a consistent awareness of and interest in significant others who are realistically perceived, empathized with, and emotionally desired or disliked or feared.

The dyadic units constituted by the representations of self and significant others, and the dominant affect framing their interactions, divide all early internalizations into affectively positive and negative ones and eventually into respectively idealized and persecutory internalized object relations. These units are the constituents of unconscious fantasy, which amplifies both expected and desired ideal relationships and the threat and trauma of aversive, painful, and frightening experiences. Positive experiences are merged into a world of ideal relationships, and negative experiences are merged into an intolerable, persecutory world.

Severely negative internalized object relations relating to traumatic and intolerable aggressive and sexual experiences remain dynamically split off from positive representations. Thus, they preserve the quality of representations of self and others framed by these negative experiences and, when excessive, prevent the eventual integration of positive and negative experiences into a whole. This permanent split related to dominance of aggression is reflected in borderline personality organization, whereas achievement of integration characterizes neurotic personality organization and normality. Normality implies an integrated self relating to integrated representations of significant others. That also applies to neurotic personality organization, but here there are rigid, restrictive character patterns in place.

The developmental aspects of affective memory accumulation vary significantly in their clinical manifestations both in health and in pathology. First, the infantile experience is conscious in terms of the activation of affective systems determining involvement in interpersonal relations; the internalization of affective dyads of self and others, both positive and negative; and the establishment of habitual behavior patterns on the basis of these early experiences, which are conscious but cannot yet be transferred into long-term memory. The effect of the earliest object relations, normal or traumatic, only remains in structured primitive behavior patterns and, perhaps, in some specific sensory perceptive effects of severe traumatization. The individual's incapacity to develop long-term memory before 2 or 3 years of age makes it impossible to retain any psychic content or conscious or unconscious emotional cognition during this time. Therefore, severe traumatization in the first few months or years of life may determine pathological patterns of behavioral interaction but without conscious or unconscious memory of their origin. This has special implications for psychotherapeutic technique.

Under ordinary circumstances, these earliest experiences merge with the second developmental stage, which involves the capacity to form long-term conscious and unconscious memory. What predominates is the dissociation between the early idealized and persecutory internalized object relations, the typical affective structures that develop during the second and third year of life. This development corresponds to what Melanie Klein described as the paranoid–schizoid position (Klein 1946). If negative and aggressive experiences predominate, idealized and persecutory internalized object relations fail to integrate, leading to fixation of a borderline personality organization—that is, of a personality organization in which splitting mechanisms and the dynamic conflicts between idealized and persecutory internalized object relations predominate. Here the affective experiences are conscious but dissociated, and interpretive psychotherapeutic interventions are geared toward resolving the dominant primitive defensive operations of splitting, projective identification, denial, primitive idealization, devaluation, and omnipotent control. All of these defensive operations interfere with the integration of a normal identity and the establishment of a neurotic and normal personality organization. This fixed dissociation constitutes "identity diffusion." This is the territory of severe personality disorders. TFP, a therapeutic approach derived from psychoanalytic object relations theory, deals specifically with these characteristics as past unresolved pathogenic conflicts are reactivated in the relationship between patient and therapist.

The third period, which predominates from the third or fourth year of life onward, is one in which idealized and persecutory internalized object relations are integrated—the depressive position in Kleinian theory. This integration applies to the development of normal identity and of repression as a dominant defensive mechanism, with the related defensive mechanisms of intellectualization, rationalization, reaction formulation, and mature forms of projection and negation. This period marks consolidation of the definite tripartite structure, in which consciousness and preconsciousness, the ego, is separated by a repressive barrier from the dynamic unconscious, the id, in its structural form. Here the psychotherapeutic technique is geared toward interpreting repression-related mechanisms to allow the repressed unconscious to emerge into consciousness.

The development of an integrated concept of the self and of significant others, both good and bad, contributes to the development of an ego ideal that also integrates the desirable aspects of an ideal self and ideal objects. By the same token, this integration also facilitates a more realistic set of internalized mandates and prohibitions, the constituents of an integrated superego in which aggression has been tamed and sexuality integrated in a tolerable way. All of these childhood processes are renewed in adolescence, with further organization of the superego and consolidation of repressive barriers against the dynamic unconscious.

Transference Analysis

Classical psychoanalytic technique involved efforts to reach pathogenic unconscious conflicts via a technical approach that invited patients to free associate, to say whatever came to mind on an ongoing basis, and clinicians to diagnose by analyzing the emergent content of patients' revealed subjective experience, both the defense mechanisms and the corresponding underlying impulses against which they had been erected. Interpretation of these defenses and their motivations facilitated the emergence into consciousness of repressed libidinal or aggressive conflictual impulses. Over time, the application of psychoanalytic technique led to the discovery that past unresolved unconscious intrapsychic conflicts emerged not only through the subjective experience communicated by patients but also, and eventually predominantly, through the behavior patterns in the therapeutic relationship that reflected these conflicts. Thus, repressed unconscious conflicts would emerge not only in the verbal content of the sessions but also in the nonverbal manifestations of motivated behaviors. Patients' interpersonal patterns in their relation with the psychoanalyst typically would evoke intense affective reactions in the analyst that would facilitate analysis of the meaning of the behavior activated in the patient. Thus, the most important manifestation of the interpretively facilitated emergence of pathogenic unconscious conflicts was their unconscious repetition in the present. That emergence in and analysis of the transference became the main source of exploration and change brought about by psychoanalytic treatment (Sandler et al. 1969).

In contemporary psychoanalytic object relations theory, awareness of the importance of the transference intensified as it became clear that unconscious conflicts were not simply conflicts between libidinal and aggressive impulses but conflicts between affectively positive invested internalized object relations and affectively negative activated internalized object relations, and that both defensive operations and the impulses they defended against were represented by idealized or persecutory internalized object relations. The transference signified the activation of repressed or dissociated internalized object relations in the form of dyadic units of self and object representations linked by a specific affect disposition. It emerged as the activation of a specific affective relationship between patient and therapist that reflected one aspect, defensive or impulsive, of a pathogenic dynamic unconscious conflict that needed to be analyzed, interpreted, and resolved. This reactivation of past experiences in the transference is not simply a reproduction of them but a combination of actual and fantasized experiences and defenses against both (Klein 1952).

The reactivation of past internalized object relations is reflected in the patient enacting the self-representation of the past conflict while projecting enactment of the object representation onto the analyst, or vice versa: the patient identifying with the object representation of the past relationship and projecting the corresponding self-representation onto the therapist. In either case, a dominant positive or negative affect would signal the specific meaning of the respective object relation activated in the transference and thus permit its clarification in the present. More generally, past unresolved intrapsychic conflicts remain active not only as dissociated or repressed memories but as highly motivated dispositions to repeat these conflicts—an unconscious effort to achieve resolution in the present that the patient was not able to achieve in the past. Libido and aggression, the supraordinate integration, respectively, of positive and negative affectively activated internalized object relations, are reproduced as their correspondent dominant affect, self-representation, and object representation. They are the content of the respective emotional-cognitive experiences in the transference.

Inappropriate present-day behaviors in interpersonal interactions that are unconsciously geared toward resolving past traumatic experiences constitute living manifestations of the unresolved past. Our general characterological dispositions, the dynamically integrated set of habitual behavior patterns that constitute our character, are powerfully influenced not only by genetic and temperamental disposition but also, most importantly, by our early interpersonal experiences. Because learning to relate to significant others is always conflictual to some extent, our present-day idiosyncratic behavior patterns represent the result of such conflictual relations in the past.

Under normal circumstances, behavioral quirks are relatively unimportant and, in ordinary social interactions, tend to be muted or neutralized. Patients with severe personality disorders, however, display these distorted patterns to a much higher extent, causing difficulties in their daily lives, work and profession, love and sex, and social life and creativity. It is precisely these distorted patterns and consequent difficulties that bring them to treatment. The dominance of these pathological behavioral patterns signifies a heightened disposition to regressive transference developments and pathological behavior patterns that will arise during treatment. This is the basic reason why transference analysis and transference resolution have become the center of the application of psychoanalytic object relations theory in the treatment of severe personality disorders.

The systematic analysis of transference developments is the road to understanding and resolving these patients' dominant past unconscious conflicts. TFP is centered on the analysis of the transference, and its main technical instruments include the interpretation of patients' behavior in treatment as it reflects activation of specific transferences and the conflicts they imply (Kernberg 2018). The activation of dominant internalized object relations is interpreted both in their defensive function, as a protection against opposite relationships that they attempt to avoid, and in their impulsive function, as an internalized object relation that reflects deeper, primitive, affectively motivated behavior that could not be satisfied in an adaptive way and constituted a permanent pressure for actualization that the patient had to defend against. Thus, the interpretation of unconsciously activated transferences, the utilization of the therapist's countertransference reactions, and the therapist's need to maintain a concerned, technically neutral objective stance are essential technical approaches in the treatment of patients with personality disorders. Transference interpretation includes clarifying the patient's subjective experience, tactfully confronting nonverbal behavior patterns, and establishing specific hypotheses regarding the meaning of the behavior in relation to the therapist. Countertransference analysis is a crucial complement to transference analysis. Major present-day conflicts that patients deny or avoid, at great risk, also may reflect the activation of the transference. In short, the dominant psychoanalytic techniques in TFP are interpretation, transference analysis, technical neutrality, and countertransference utilization.

Analysis of the transference demands a "normal" therapeutic frame against which the activation of transference behavior can be evaluated. Patients are encouraged to free associate, a specific therapeutic requirement that must be explicitly described as their dominant task. They are encouraged to express themselves freely within the ordinary boundaries of a psychotherapeutic relationship. The therapist clarifies his or her own role in interpreting the deeper meanings of what emerges during sessions as he or she is able to express them to patients and help them deepen their own understanding. Certain limits and arrangements for how sessions will be conducted may be set according to specific psychopathologies because the patient's life, health, and relationships may be threatened by the severity of some transference regressions. The therapist must remain alert to emergent transference through combined analysis of the free association, the nonverbal communication, and the countertransference. A first step in this endeavor is being alert to any significant deviations from the optimal behavior of the patient's task (free association) or the therapist's task (interpretation) and to what is affectively dominant.

Affective dominance refers to what, in the overall impression of the therapist, is most strongly present at any moment of the session as affectively implied by the various behavioral components (Caligor et al. 2018). Sometimes what is affectively dominant is something that happened outside the sessions that the patient describes with intense affect or a memory that the patient refers to. At other times, a development in the therapist's countertransference may become dominant and must be analyzed regarding its relation to the patient in the session. Sometimes an idiosyncratic behavior pattern that develops in parallel to what the patient is discussing becomes affectively dominant in terms of the therapist's experience. Learning to assess what is affectively dominant is an important task for the therapist and goes hand-in-hand with the parallel task of identifying the specific object relationship that the affective dominance represents. Once a dominant affective relationship is defined as such, assessing who is enacting the role of the patient's self and who is enacting the role of the corresponding object becomes clearer.

Not everything is transference. The intense emotional reaction of patients to certain behaviors or lack of behaviors on the part of the therapist may reflect a transference reaction or be a realistic response to an inappropriate behavior on the therapist's part. Patients' protests against therapists' behavior must be carefully explored within the reality of the complaint, and therapists must not only be honest in exploring their own behavior but be able to acknowledge objective causes for the patient's protest. Such incidents should be addressed without excessive defensiveness or guilt but with truthfulness and maintaining the technical neutrality that reflects an objective concern for the patient. It is a subtle, consistent task for therapists to maintain their side of the "normal" therapeutic relationship.

At the same time, what is affectively dominant may have to do with the patient's relationship with other persons outside of the therapeutic relationship rather than with the therapist. However, transference developments are most often defended against through projection onto other persons or situations outside of the treatment situation itself. The concept of "total transference" refers to including in the transference analysis not only developments that evolve in free association but also those related to events occurring outside the session that may, at first, seem to have no relation to the patient–therapist interaction (Joseph 1985).

Often, what begins as the analysis of the emotional implication of a conflict the patient has with an outside person or situation rapidly turns into an affectively dominant issue in the transference. Two relatively common defensive operations against awareness of a conflict in the transference are acting out and somatization. *Acting out* refers to the expression of the patients' conflict through determined actions rather than emotional awareness. Patients act out in behavior what they cannot consciously tolerate. Somatic reactions during the sessions, physical expressions of anxiety and depression, or specific conversion symptoms may evolve during moments when the emotional aspects of a transference reaction cannot be tolerated. Under these circumstances, both acting out and somatization must be translated into the emotional transferential situation the patient is avoiding.

Sometimes the nature of patients' physical or emotional symptoms or of their difficulties with significant others seems so distant from anything evolving in the therapeutic relationship that it seems doubtful that any transference development is taking place. Discovery of the link between the outside issues and the relationship with the therapist may take time and may emerge unexpectedly following the analysis of a particular transference aspect. With some experience, therapists discover that the absence of an apparent transference *is* the transference. This is most frequently an aspect of the particular pathology of narcissistic personality disorders. Narcissistic transferences are characterized by patients' difficulty accepting an authentic dependence on the therapist. Patients maintain a friendly or noncommittal "objectivity" in their relationship with the therapist that reflects this incapacity to depend. TFP has developed specific techniques to deal with this difficulty that not only are effective but have an important function in the fundamental resolution of severe narcissistic pathology (Kernberg 2018).

An effective way to defend against transference regression and, in fact, to defend against the emergence of a dominant transference reaction is demonstrated by the patient who transforms free association into an ongoing dialogue with the therapist that maintains the therapeutic relationship at a superficial level. Observing patients' capacity or lack of capacity to carry out free association, tolerating periods of silence while patients affirm that nothing is going on in their mind or recite a litany of surface complaints with no attempt to explore or understand them, and tolerating silences and pregnant moments in which verbal communication is not available are all important features in the challenge of diagnosing the dominant activated transference disposition. The patient's difficulty with freely floating communication about his or her subjective experience is already an indication that something is interfering with the patient's ability to relate to the therapist.

Transference developments may be classified into various dominant types. The traditional reference to positive and negative transferences is of little practical help; however, the awareness of certain typical characterological styles in the transference is relevant for the systematic analysis of transference resistances. For example, in paranoid transferences, intense distrust, hypersensitivity, and negative affects predominate. Depressive transferences are characterized by intense feelings of guilt, depressive reactions, and experience of the therapist as a strict and harsh authority. In "psychopathic" transferences, the patient believes the therapist is not being honest or the patient is dishonest or deceptive. Narcissistic transferences are characterized by an enormous emotional distance and an apparent lack of development or specific affective reactions in the relationship with the therapist. Schizoid transferences involve a significant fragmentation of the patient's affective experience, an enormous chaos of self-experience. In "symbiotic" transferences, patients only tolerate the therapist's total agreement with their feelings or thoughts and experience any independent thinking on the part of the therapist as a brutal attack, invasion, or abandonment. Finally, in severely aggressive psychotic transferences, ordinary reality testing is lost; hallucinations or delusions may evolve or patients may be completely confused as to whether their ideas and feelings stem from the therapist or themselves. The diagnosis of and particular therapeutic approaches to these various transferences is an important aspect of TFP technique. An awareness of these major types helps the therapist diagnose conditions when transference developments are characterized by a dominant transference that colors every particular activation of a specific object relation in the transference (Kernberg 2020).

In conclusion, contemporary psychoanalytic object relations theory explains the development of significant structural organization of psychic experience under conditions of normality and pathology, points to the basic nature of the dyadic units of self-object-affect units, and helps to clarify the function of these internalized object relations both as defensive and impulsive processes. Conflicts between contradictory internalized object relations that are activated in the transference constitute the clinical manifestation of pathogenic unconscious intrapsychic conflicts. Analysis in the transference of these activated internalized object relations, clarifying their self and object components, and the reciprocal activation of these components within the frame of the dominant affect in the patient's relation with the therapist constitutes transference analysis, the dominant technical approach in TFP.

References

Caligor E, Kernberg OF, Clarkin JF, Yeomans FE: Psychodynamic Therapy for Personality Pathology: Treating Self and Interpersonal Functioning. Washington, DC, American Psychiatric Association Publishing, 2018

Joseph B: Transference: the total situation. Int J Psychoanal 66:447–454, 1985

Kernberg OF: Resolution of Aggression and Recovery of Eroticism. Washington, DC, American Psychiatric Association Publishing, 2018

Kernberg OF: Therapeutic implications of transference structures in various personality pathologies. J Am Psychoanal Assoc 67:951–986, 2020

Kernberg OF: Some Implications of New Developments in Neurobiology for Psychoanalytic Object Relations Theory. Unpublished manuscript, 2021

Klein M: Notes on some schizoid mechanisms. Int J Psychoanal 27:99–110, 1946

Klein M: The origins of transference. Int J Psychoanal 33:433–438, 1952

Sandler J, Holders A, Kawenoka M, et al: Notes on some theoretical and clinical aspects of transference. Int J Psychoanal 50:633–645, 1969

Yeomans F, Clarkin JF, Kernberg OF: Transference Focused Psychotherapy for Borderline Personality Disorders: A Clinical Guide. Washington, DC, American Psychiatric Publishing, 2015

CHAPTER 2

Some Implications of New Developments in Neurobiology for Psychoanalytic Object Relations Theory

Drives and Affects

What follows is my understanding of changes in psychoanalytic theory and its application to standard psychoanalysis and psychoanalytic psychotherapies as suggested by new developments both in neurobiology and psychoanalytic object relations theory. Specifically, I believe psychoanalytic theory needs to be revised in two major areas: 1) the theory of drives, and 2) the theory of the dynamic unconscious.

From Kernberg OF: "Some Implications of New Developments in Neurobiology for Psychoanalytic Object Relations Theory." *Neuropsychoanalysis*, 2021. Published online November 25, 2021. DOI: 10.1080/15294145.2021.1995609. Copyright © 2021 The International Neuropsychoanalysis Society, reprinted by permission of Taylor & Francis Ltd. (http://www.tandfonline.com) on behalf of The International Neuropsychoanalysis Society.

Neurobiological Evidence: Affect Systems as Primary Motivators

To begin with, the psychoanalytic theory of drives needs significant revision. Freud had proposed that the basic motivational systems of psychic functioning were libido and the death drive, or libido and aggression (Freud 1915/1957, 1923/1961). Freud located the origin of the libidinal drive in the erotogenic zones of the skin and related mucous membranes, described in detail the development of sexual drive from multiple, polymorphous sexual impulses and their integration into the dominance of genital sexuality, and related these developments of libido to the culmination of their corresponding object relations in the oedipal constellation. He had not described, however, the origin and development of the death drive or aggression. The ultimate purpose of "Nirvana" or self-destruction as the objective of the aggressive drive has remained as a controversial aspect of the classical dual drive theory.

I believe that while the clinical relevance of unconscious conflicts between libidinal and aggressive impulses remain the fundamental etiology common to all unconscious conflicts, the origin of the corresponding neurotic and characterological pathology, and an important aspect of psychotic pathology as well, the present-day neurobiological evidence points to the affect systems as the primary motivators of human behavior (Kernberg 2004a, 2006). I believe that the contemporary classification of affect systems into positive ones: attachment, erotism, and play bonding—and negative ones: fight-flight and separation-panic—covers the development of essential psychic motivation from beginning of life to their most complex derivatives (Panksepp 1998; Panksepp and Biven 2012). There is ample empirical evidence for the brain structures and neurotransmitters of these affect systems and for their functions in activating behavior as well as specific subjective experience (Damasio 2010; Krause 2012). I have proposed that the division of affect systems into positive and negative ones signals the potential for the integration, respectively, of the positive affect systems as a major overall drive—libido—and the integrative consolidation of the negative affect systems into an overall drive: aggression (Kernberg 2004a, 2004b, 2006). The basis for this classification is the originally pleasurable affiliative quality of the "positive" affect systems, in contrast to the opposite, painfully disaffiliative or antagonistic quality of the "negative" affect systems.

Thus, libido and aggression emerge as the developmentally supraordinate integration of these component affective systems. The positive affect systems of attachment, erotism, and play bonding give origin, respectively, to the fundamental motivational drive of dependency, sexuality, and affiliative interaction that, jointly, constitute libido. They all include appetitive ("longing") and consummatory pleasures. The analysis of the concept of libido throughout all psychoanalytic writings illustrates these libidinal components: the search for dependency and its conflicts related to fears of abandonment; the desires of sexuality and the conflicts derived from basic oedipal desire and prohibitions, rivalry, and guilt; and the search for personal friendship and community participation in conflict with interpersonal competition and self-affirmation. The negative affect systems, namely, fight-flight and separation-panic, signal the major components of what will be integrated as the aggressive drive, including the aggressive effort to combat and destroy dangerous, damaging, threatening objects or situations, and the efforts to escape from dangerous situations that cannot be overcome or eliminated. The emergency affective system of separation-panic emerges as the emotional reaction to an immediate threat to physical or psychological survival that separation from caregivers represents for young animals, as well as the effort to escape or deny an intolerable, life-threatening reality. Finally, the additional, primary affective "SEEKING" system represents a general affective disposition to explore the environment and to reinforce the approach to gratifying objects or situations.

We now know the brain networks involved in the activation and control of these affective systems (Panksepp 1998; Panksepp and Biven 2012). The activation of the respective affective experiences and affect-driven behavior extends across a wide spectrum of brainstem and limbic areas of the brain. The activation of consciousness and focused alertness to reality arises in the brainstem, and the cognitive contextualization and control related to affects resides in cortical areas of the brain (Roth 2001; Roth and Strüber 2014).

Affects constitute the organism's basic motivation to adapt to its environment, protect the homeostasis of essential biological requirements, react to sources of pain and pleasure, and, at the higher psychological level of this adaptive effort, regulate the internal and external relations with significant others. At a basic brainstem level, affects have a homeostatic function that usually does not reach consciousness, such as the control of temperature, blood circulation, and breathing. Some of these homeostatic mechanisms do break into consciousness in emergencies (hypothermia, suffocation). Conscious levels of affect activation are determined by sensorial stimuli that determine the experience of sensorial displeasure or pain or by cognitive assessment of predicted pain or pleasure. These stimuli are processed in cortical regions and widely distributed through the brain. Sensorial experience is an originally unconscious cortical function that evolves into a conscious experience only after transfer into the associative cortical region. However, pain, a sensory affect, seems to be generated at the level of the PAG in the midbrain.

At higher levels of limbic structures—in mesencephalic and diencephalic brain structures—the activation of affective needs in relation to other, human objects dominate desires that link the organism with its immediate psychosocial environment. The affective linkage between the emerging self and its significant human objects represents the highest limbic level, connecting midbrain and other subcortical structures with the associative cortex. The associative cortex elaborates the conscious experience of affects as a central constituent of the self and of the representations of others. Here, affective experience is amplified by cortical functions that integrate consciously sensorial experience, its cognitive framing, and the developing capacity for long-term memory into the conscious, self-aware aspects of experience of emotion. The psychosocial contextual environment, originally, the baby–mother relationship, is internalized as the double aspect of emotional experience and awareness of this experience as self-experience, in parallel to the attribution of similar emotional experience to mother or the significant other. Gradually the experience of others is perceived as willful behavior, with growing empathy by the self, and, eventually, a realistic awareness of the minds of others as well as highly individualized emotional investments in significant others (Förstl 2012). This process represents the neurobiological basis for the development of intrapsychic dyadic structures, experiential units of self-representation affectively linked to an object representation, the "building blocks" of the mind, the components of unconscious fantasy (Northoff 2011).

In my view, the function of affect systems to relate the individual to one's psychosocial environment may be considered the most remarkable development of the human psyche. The highest level of the limbic system combines the expression of specific affects in intimate relationships with the cognitive functions of the associative cortical areas. This process culminates in the function of the "working memory," which includes the development of an integrated concept of self, that is, an integrated view of the individual placed in time and space, with authority of movement, utilization of memory, and awareness of emotional needs to relate to selective significant others. By the same token, this process includes the parallel construction of an internal world of significant others and their assumed—and gradually more realistically assessed—emotional reality (Svrakic and Divac-Jovanovic 2019).

The Representations of Self and Others

The concept of self includes an autobiographical awareness, together with imagination and planning in the context of a consistent awareness and interest in significant others, again, realistically perceived, empathized with, and emotionally desired. In my view (Kernberg 2018; Northoff et al. 2016; Roth and Strüber 2014), the ventromedial preorbital and prefrontal cortex, the anterior part of the cingulum, the insula, and widespread areas within the parietal and temporal lobe all are involved predominantly in this synthetic function of the self, while, in parallel, the dorsolateral aspects of the prefrontal cortex, the parietal-temporal junction, and numerous additional lateral cortical areas focus mostly on the nature of the human other, and the self-relation to the objects of one's search and desires and fears. Essentially, an organization of emotional experiences defining the relationship between self and others evolves and is internalized as affective memories. Repeated in thousands of interactions from birth on, affective memory is internalized as a central function of the hippocampus as the "memory chamber" (Roth and Dicke 2006). A neural network related to this hippocampus function will evaluate the positive or negative potential of any new experience with significant others, and fundamentally contribute, together with the associative cortex, to the buildup of an internal world of object relations, conscious and unconscious (more about this to follow) (Svrakic and Divac-Jovanovic 2019).

As I have previously proposed (see, e.g., Kernberg 2001, 2012), the dyadic units constituted by the representation of self, the representation of a significant other, and a dominant affect framing their interaction divide all early internalizations into affectively positive and affectively negative ones, and, eventually, into respectively idealized and persecutory internal object relations. These units are the constituents of unconscious fantasy. As such, they remain as deep layers of affective memories in the hippocampus and other affective and procedural memory circuits. We know from the neurobiology of affect activation, as well as from the observation of infants and small children, that positive and negative units of experience are originally split, dissociated from each other, while all the positive experiences tend to be merged as a world of ideal relationships, and all the negative, in parallel, will merge as an intolerable, persecutory world. I propose that the later, integrative gathering of these experiences, their modulating and more realistic integration, is a function of the associative cortex, linked to the elaboration of emotional experiences in consciousness (Kernberg 2012; Northoff et al. 2016). I further suggest that prefrontal, preorbital, circulate, and insular cortical functions integrate the originally split "good" and "bad" concepts of self and significant others, leading to realistic total object relations and corresponding neurotic and normal personality structure.

Severely conflictual, intolerable internalized object relations that remain dynamically split preserve the quality of representations of self and others framed by extreme affects and unconsciously are either extremely desired or feared. They become the constituents of the dynamic unconscious.

I believe that this concept of self-object-affect relations as positive and negative building blocks of the mind corresponds to the nature of unconscious fantasy as described by the Kleinian psychoanalytic school (Isaacs 1948; Spillius et al. 2011). I believe that each unconscious fantasy is, at bottom, a highly desired or terribly feared unit of an embedded self/object representation relationship and the correspondent affect, reflecting a consciously intolerable fantasy.

The activation of these internalized object relations in the transference between patient and therapist in intensive psychodynamic treatment constitutes the dominant expression of the unresolved conflictual unconscious past. The analysis of transference is represented by the analysis of the corresponding activation of representations of self and other and of the dominant affect linking them expressing the desired or feared interaction. The respective representation of the object may be projected onto the therapist while the corresponding representation of self is enacted by the patient (prevalent with neurotic personality organization), or, with rapid interchange of roles in the case of borderline personality organization, the patient may enact an identification with the object while the corresponding self-representation is projected onto the therapist. Transference interpretation is an analysis of the dominant, consciously activated dyadic units, in the context of the simultaneous maintenance of an external perspective, the therapist's interpretive function as an "excluded other," a triangulation that facilitates the patient's insight and the development of his emotional capacity to tolerate such a triangular vision himself (Yeomans et al. 2015).

So far, I have pointed to a significant shift in the concept of motivational systems, from Freud's original dual drive theory to an affect theory of motivation that conceives drives as a supraordinate, second level of development. Drives, thus conceived, become activated in the clinical situation in their component affect dispositions and related object relations. This conception of drives corresponds closely with the contemporary concept of psychoanalytic object relations theory. In my view, it does not replace the dual concept of drives proposed by Freud but puts them into the context of a primary motivational system of affects that reflects our present knowledge of the neurobiological determinants of psychic life. Clinically, unconscious conflict is mainly still between love and aggression.

The Death Drive

Freud's theory of the death drive was based upon his clinical observations of severe forms of self-destructive psychopathology, including repetition compulsion, sadism/masochism, negative therapeutic reaction, suicide in severe depression and in non-depressive characterological structures, and destructive and self-destructive developments in group processes and their social implications (Kernberg 2009). In the light of today's experience, regarding both the diagnosis and treatment of severe forms of psychopathology and the reality of social conflicts under conditions of the mass psychology of the last 100 years, Freud's observations regarding self-directed aggression have been dramatically confirmed. In all of these areas in which Freud described the importance of self-directed and potentially deadly aggression, we have found that analysis of the psychodynamics of the intrapsychic development of borderline conditions, or, respectively, the ideological preconditions for the development of severe social self-destructiveness, all indicate that such severe self-directed aggression is a pathological consequence of an excessive predominance of negative affect systems. In other words, in contrast to the normal predominance of positive affective systems under conditions of relatively normal psychological developments from birth on, particularly in the first few years of life, a predominance of a severely negative, aggressive disposition is a fundamental causal factor of these severe psychopathologies. Excessive negative affect systems may be the consequence of genetic, constitutional, and temperamental factors in some cases, but environmental causes predominate in the large majority of types of pathology that direct aggression against the self. Insecure attachment; exposure to physical, emotional, or sexual abuse; early abandonment; and chronically chaotic family situations reinforced by further significant deprivation, aggressive and sexual traumatization during childhood and early adolescence are major causes of self-directed aggression (Kernberg 2004b).

André Green (1993, 2007) first pointed to the fact that Freud's concept of the death drive reflected his awareness of what Green called "negative narcissism," namely, the fact that the investment of the self-structure is not only with libido or positive affect systems but also with a certain amount of negative affect systems, a potential for fight and aggressive self-affirmation that is part of the normal development of autonomy, self-affirmation, resilience, and dealing with the ambivalent features of ordinary social life. It is only under conditions of severe traumatization, in psychopathological developments, that what originally was a positive, functional investment of aggression by the self (together with the identification of the self with predominant libidinal, positive affect systems), now would become what Freud called the death drive. In simple terms, the death drive is a secondary motivational system that reflects the pathological, exaggerated self-directed investment with negative affect systems that, under ordinary conditions, are mostly directed outside the self.

The Dynamic Unconscious

In addition to the concept of drives, another major concept of classical psychoanalysis that requires revision is that of the dynamic unconscious. The prevalence of unconscious processes in psychic development has been amply confirmed. However, the structure of the unconscious and its dominant influences on consciousness needs to be reformulated, in my view.

Recent neurobiological findings indicate that consciousness and unconsciousness evolve in parallel from the beginning of life (Roth and Strüber 2014). Unconsciousness may be divided into the "primary unconscious," which includes the functions of all subcortical brain regions and the non-associative cortical functions, and the "secondary unconscious," that refers to the cumulative emotional processes of the infant and the small child before maturation of the associative cortex. The secondary unconscious also includes unconscious "procedural memory," the early learning of skills that, after initial conscious experience, become automatic and persist in unconscious behaviors. This early learning, however, also includes learning of ways to relate self to the environment, determining the earliest and potentially very influential structures of self and representations of significant others that, while originally conscious, because of the early lack of maturation of the capacity for long-term memory (that only develops, during the second and third year of life, with the maturation of the associative cortex and the hippocampus) are erased from conscious memory or may never have been recorded declaratively (Solms 2015).

I believe that these earliest learning processes affect behavior in the form of unconscious procedural memory, but without reaching the long-term "dynamic unconscious," nor ever being available to consciousness because they leave no trace other than that immediately activated and learned behavior. In addition, during the entire childhood development, consciously learned activities, integration between sensorial and motor processes, may remain as procedural memory and sink into unconsciousness: for example, learning how to ride a bicycle or how to play the piano.

At the point when the development of long-term memory becomes available, around the end of the second and in the course of third year of life, with the maturation of the hippocampus as "affective memory storage facility" and the development of the associative cortex, conscious experiences may now become dynamically unconscious and constitute the dynamic unconscious proper. Thus, the dynamic unconscious is linked to the capacity for long-term declarative memory because, according to my view, by definition the content of the dynamic unconscious was originally conscious and has become repressed or dissociated in the course of development. Broadly speaking, then, the unconscious includes both procedural, unconscious memory and explicit, episodic, declarative memory. However, only the latter is the basis of the dynamic unconscious proper. To repeat, all subcortical brain regions and non-associative cortical brain regions constitute the primary unconscious. The affective processes and emotional experiences of infant and small child before the maturation of the associative cortex and hippocampus leave significant behavioral traces, but no memory, and only later, repressed and dissociated experiences determine the dynamic unconscious.

It is important to point out that, as mentioned earlier, all sensorial stimuli are originally unconscious and only selectively enter into consciousness after a very fast and complex selective, unconscious cortical and subcortical process that determines the input into the associative cortical area, that is, consciousness (Le Doux 2019). All sensorial stimuli are widely distributed to various brain regions and systematically explored (in 300 milliseconds) for their newness, significance, positive or negative affective value, with input from the sensorial thalamic system and affect-activating limbic structures such as the ventral tegmental area, the nucleus accumbens, and activating amygdala. The hippocampus and dorsal striatum are also involved in the decision-making process regarding which stimuli are to become conscious. All sensorial perceptions selected to become conscious are channeled through the thalamus, which acts as a "port of entry and exit" into cortical consciousness (Roth 2001). Consciousness is originally determined at the inferior limbic level, particularly the periaqueductal gray, reticular formation, locus coeruleus, and raphe nuclei. It is activated by the basic affective systems such as the sensorial reaction to pain and, most importantly, by homeostatic requirements of temperature, blood circulation, hunger, and thirst (Roth and Strüber 2014). In the first year of life, consciousness emerges by the activation of any and all of the major affect systems involving the interpersonal world that I outlined above (Roth 2014).

Eventually, human consciousness involves the awareness of self, of one's body, one's placement of self and body in space and time, the experience of one's identity and its autobiographical continuity, the function of one's actions and mental acts, and, gradually, the differentiation of reality and imagination. These are background features of the self that converge in consciousness and depend on the integration of information from multiple brain regions, including, particularly, the posterior cingulate cortex, the posterior parietal cortex, and the dorsal lateral prefrontal cortex, that constitutes the "working memory" of actual consciousness. Working memory includes, in addition to all of the above-mentioned aspects of awareness, one's present awareness of the environment of one's body, one's present awareness of needs, affects, and emotions, and one's focused attention on specific aspects of one's relationship with the environment, as well as the general functions of thinking, imagining, and remembering. In short, consciousness includes fundamentally the consciousness of self, its expectations, desires, and fears, and its assessment of the psychosocial environment, that is, the nature of and relationship with others and the mutual influence of self and others in their interaction.

In parallel with the building up of the structure of the self, the structure of significant others is built up on the basis of cognitive awareness, the development of other limbic structures that originate the capacity for empathy, theory of mind, and the direct affective and cognitive interaction with others (Förstl 2012). I have already referred to the corresponding functions of the dorsolateral prefrontal cortex and would add here the important role of the insula and the parietal-temporal junction.

Thus, I believe the unconscious is even more important in determining human experience and behavior than Freud assumed, including the procedural memory unconscious that derives from sensorial and motor experiences and the long-term procedural memory derived from automated learning. The declarative memory unconscious, that is, the unconscious that contains both explicit memory episodes and semantic memory, permits the development of the dynamic unconscious, which, I now suggest, may be divided developmentally into three major timespans.

Developmental Phases of the Dynamic Unconscious

First, the infantile experience, from birth on, is conscious in terms of the activation of affect systems determining the involvement in interpersonal relations, and habitual behavior patterns are established based on these early experiences that are conscious but that cannot yet be transferred into long-term declarative memory. This early time corresponds to the normal infantile amnesia. In addition, this period is the beginning of the internalization of affective dyads of self and others (Hart 2008; Kernberg 2012; Stern 1985). Thus the effect of the earliest object relations, normal or traumatic, only remains in temperamental and primitive behavior patterns, and perhaps in some specific effects of traumatization (Coates et al. 2003). In this regard, Freud was wrong regarding the unconscious origin of the dynamic unconscious. As Mark Solms (2015) first pointed out, based on modern affect theory, particularly Panksepp's contributions, the dynamic unconscious is originally conscious. The ego, insofar as we consider the establishment of habitual behavior patterns as part of the control system of the ego, is originally unconscious in terms of learned patterns that at times may reflect significant traumatic experiences that left no mental content.

The second developmental period involves the development of the capacity for long-term conscious and unconscious declarative memory, with a predominance of dissociation between idealized and persecutory internalized object relations that are the typical affective structures that develop in the second and third year of life. This development corresponds to the psychodynamics Melanie Klein described as the "paranoid-schizoid position" (Klein 1946). As I have described in detail elsewhere (Kernberg 2001, 2012), if negative and aggressive experiences predominate, the integration of idealized and persecutory internalized object relations fails to take place, leading to the fixation of borderline personality organization—that is, fixation of an organization of the personality with a predominance of splitting operations of the dynamic conflicts between idealized and persecutory internalized object relations. Here the affective experiences are conscious but dissociated, in the moment, from other experiences. In treatment, interpretive interventions are geared to resolving the dominant primitive defensive operations (splitting, projective identification, denial, primitive idealization, devaluation, and omnipotent control) that interfere with the integration of normal identity and the setting up of a neurotic and normal personality structure (Yeomans et al. 2015).

Lastly, the third period that predominates from the third or fourth year of life is a period of integration of idealized and persecutory internalized object relations, the "depressive position" (Klein 1946), resulting in the development of normal identity and of repression as the dominant defensive mechanism, with the related defensive mechanisms of intellectualization, rationalization, reaction formation, and mature forms of projection and negation. This period of development marks the consolidation of the tripartite structure, in which the consciousness and preconsciousness, i.e., the ego, are separated by a repressive barrier from the dynamic unconscious, or what we might call the id in its *mature* form. Here, the psychotherapeutic technique is to interpret repression and related mechanisms to permit the emergence of the repressed unconscious into consciousness (Kernberg 2018).

Therapeutic Implications

This outline of the developmental phases of unconscious mental conflict has diagnostic and therapeutic implications. The predominance of extremely traumatic circumstances in the first year or two of life would not leave unconscious representations of self and object representations, only extreme dispositions to negative affect with potential fragmentation of affect experience to escape the panic-separation system. These traumatic psychological experiences may also lead to lasting influences on neurobiological systems and brain functioning (Heim and Nemeroff 2001). These patients evince a profound disposition to behavioral pathology that emerges as bizarre interactions in the transference, the typical developments of extremely schizoid structures. The therapist may experience the implications, in the "here and now," of these pathological developments and approximate the reconstruction of what Bollas (1989) called "unthought" thoughts or experience that have to be deduced from later, secondary developments of these experiences. It implies an extremely slow and tentative work in the transference and a very important utilization of countertransference reactions.

Clinical experiences with severely schizoid and schizophrenic individuals have indicated very primitive mechanisms of fragmentation of affective experience geared to reduce the attention to and investment in the external world, with the danger of confusion between good and bad experiences in the interpersonal field, a general withdrawal from contacts, and profound distrust of any interpersonal experience (Rosenfeld 1950). Severely schizoid personality structures may require particular therapeutic approaches. Under the worst circumstances, in conditions with a severe cognitive failure, a lack of differentiation between self and others may result in the loss of reality testing and a predisposition to psychosis (Dammann and Kernberg 2019).

Much more frequently, severe traumatization and pathology of aggression affect the second level of development, the stage between 2 and 5 years of age, in which splitting mechanisms predominate, fostering a potential fixation at this stage that results in borderline personality organization. Here, the severity of negative affect activation in the form of persecutory internalized object relations that predominate over positive ones still permits the establishment of split-off positive relationships. It is likely that both genetically determined differences in neurotransmitter systems sensitizing the individual excessively to negative experiences, and hyperactivity of the amygdala or other negative affect activating structures, constitute temperamental predispositions to excessive aggressive reactions, although traumatizing early object experiences are leading etiological factors. Here idealized and persecutory internalized object relations clearly predominate and are activated in the typical transferences of borderline patients, and interpretive psychotherapeutic work focuses particularly on splitting operations, projective identification, denial, and other related, primitive defensive operations. Oedipal and pre-oedipal conflicts are combined in many ways, with aggressive object relations and affects prevalent in both areas (Kernberg 2018).

When the pathology predominates at the third level of intrapsychic organization, which involves the integration of idealized and persecutory segments of experience, the development of normal identity and mature defenses prevail. The dynamic unconscious in its "mature form" dominates. Unconscious fantasies reflect the conflicts between desired and dreaded relationships, with the accent on typical oedipal conflicts but a relative decrease of the intensity of their aggressive implications.

Now ideal self and ideal object representations are integrated into the ego ideal as part of an integrated superego, in which primitive sadistic precursors from early stages of development and later oedipal prohibitions are integrated as well. The tripartite structure of ego, superego, and id reflects this overall integration. Pathology here involves the typical symptomatic neuroses and character pathology at the level of neurotic personality organization.

The development of an integrated concept of the self, both good and bad, and of an integrated concept of significant others, both good and bad, contributes to the development of an ego ideal that also integrates the desirable aspects of an ideal self and ideal objects. By the same token, this integration also facilitates a more realistic set of internalized mandates and prohibitions, in other words, the constituents of a more mature superego, in which aggression has been tamed and sexuality integrated in a tolerable way (Jacobson 1964). All of these processes are renewed at the time of adolescence, with the further organization of the superego as well as the consolidation of the repressive barrier against the dynamic unconscious.

The general implication is that ordinary personality development starts with the internalization of dyadic object relations and splitting mechanisms and only evolves gradually into the definite structure of ego (probably better called the self at this point), the repressed dynamic unconscious, and the superego as an internalized system of integrated values. The earliest schizoid stage, under extremely traumatic conditions, with affective fragmentation and psychosocial withdrawal would reflect, if defensively fixated, the earliest psychopathology of the personality structure.

Throughout this developmental sequence, it emerges that the organization of the self, its degree of integration or splitting, constitutes a fundamental structure influencing the consolidation of habitual behavior patterns or character traits, with the understanding that the very earliest behavior patterns are determined before the existence of an integrated self and before the possibility of mentalization of earliest traumatic experiences. It is of interest that the parallel development of integrated concepts of significant others has aroused less attention on the part of neurobiologists than the analysis of the sequential development of the components of the self-structure. From the clinical viewpoint of the study of subjective intrapsychic experience reflected in unconscious fantasy, the nature of the internalized world of object relations including the sequential development of the representation of significant others is as important as that of the self. It is the relationship *between* self and significant others that one might consider as the most important intrapsychic structures influencing organization of behavior, and subjective emotional experiences—from ecstasy to despair—throughout life. I believe it is fair to say that psychoanalysis, after Freud, has neglected the study of the neurobiological roots of intrapsychic, subjective psychological structures. By the same token, neurobiology has neglected the study of the establishment of an internal world of object relations as the ultimate, most advanced objective of neurobiological developments, the autonomous dynamics of this intrapsychic world, and the fact that personality structure and functions depend on the interaction of both neurobiological and psychodynamic developments. Melanie Klein (1946; Isaacs 1948) described unconscious fantasy as the basic structures of the internal world, the product of the interaction of the mental representations of drives and early defensive operations, constituted by internalized objects and self-aspects as well as the affective derivatives of drives. This formulation corresponds, I believe, to the components of the basic dyadic structures of self-representation, object representation, and a specific affect defining their positive or negative values described by contemporary object relations theory. Herein lies a key linkage between neurobiological and psychodynamic determinants of psychic life.

This leads us to the therapeutic implications of what has been said so far in terms of the theory of unconscious conflicts, the unconscious dynamics of psychopathology, and the objective of psychoanalytic treatment. First of all, the most severe cases of early distortions of the personality are related to severe traumatization in the first year of life, probably primarily traumatization in the context of insecure attachment, with its corresponding failure of normative development of affective experience, control, and integration. Traumatic physical mistreatment; sexual mistreatment; severe, painful illness; abandonment; and chronic unpredictability of care relate to such extreme severity of illness. Here the transference will not reflect clearly any particular interactions between self and other, of which no memory remains, but rather, enacted behavior patterns derived from such early states of development. Strangely chaotic transferences may develop: emotional unavailability, the emergence of separation-panic, and primitive aggression may characterize transference developments and permit the therapist to tentatively interpret the dominant meaning of a certain object relationship in the transference in terms of a hypothetical earliest experience of life. This is, I believe, what Ogden (1997) called the "autistic-touching" earliest stage of development and what other authors have interpreted as the basic schizoid dilemma, requiring an intense, although thoughtfully managed countertransference utilization in interpreting such primitive mental states (Dammann and Kernberg 2015).

It is generally stated that these are "pre-symbolic" emotional experiences that predate the development of organized language and the capacity for symbolic thinking. However, clinically, those patients usually are both able to think and talk in ordinary ways at other moments of their daily existence, and one may question to what extent a defensive regression has taken place in the transference, which needs to be interpreted as such, and the extent to which earliest experiences may be translated into symbolic interpretation that does justice to their present reactivated affective nature. Gerhard Roth (personal communication) has suggested that purely cognitive approaches to deep-seated emotional conflicts will not be adequate because of the lack of direct limbic communication between the dorsolateral region of the prefrontal and preorbital cortex, in contrast to the effectiveness of interventions that have an important affective component, and thus relate to the ventromedial prefrontal and preorbital cortex and anterior part of the cingulum, thus reaching the deeper levels of affective experiences in the hippocampus. I have described a related technical approach with schizoid personalities in earlier work. The therapy is structured to allow for affect expression in the context of a safe environment, where the therapist is alert to assist in the patient's growing capacity to understand and modulate the affective links between self and others.

Regarding the treatment of patients with borderline personality organization, transference-focused psychotherapy (Yeomans et al. 2015) has proven to be an effective application of psychoanalytic technique, with the specific strategies and tactics required by these patients, and modified according to the predominant characterological structure that patients with borderline personality organization present (Caligor et al. 2018). Thus, borderline personality disorder, narcissistic personality disorder, and schizoid personality disorder all require modifications in the psychoanalytic technique derived from the rapid activation of role reversals of dyadic relationships, in which patient and therapist alternatively enact representation of self and other under the dominance of a predetermined primitive affect. The treatment of these conditions requires a technique different from standard psychoanalysis due to intense behavioral manifestations of primitive affective activation, lack of tolerance of emotional thinking vs. behavioral acting out, and the need to protect the structure of the treatment from severe acting out. Standard psychoanalysis, in turn, is indicated for patients with severe character pathology and regressive developments in the context of an integrated identity, a consolidated self, and stable internalized relations with significant others. The typical neurotic patient may count on psychoanalysis as the most effective treatment for neurotic syndromes and character disorders (Caligor et al. 2018; Kernberg 2018).

Conclusion

In short, psychoanalytic theory requires the following revisions:

1. The proposal that the primary motivational systems are affect systems and that libido and aggression represent secondary developments of

affect integration. Drives still derive ultimately from neurobiology but are organized and represented in unconscious conflicts between love and aggression expressed in internalized, affect invested object relations.

2. Conflicts between love and aggression are originally conscious, in the context of the primary activation of affect systems in the relation between self and other (mother), but their traces remain only in behavior patterns and fragmented affects, if extremely traumatic circumstances prevail. If less severe, these conflicts are assimilated into the second stage of splitting mechanisms and borderline personality organization. Here mutual dissociation between idealized and persecutory object relations dominates.

3. In the advance toward identity integration, repressive mechanisms and consolidations of the tripartite structure (originally, ego, superego, id) evolve, with a truly consolidated dynamic unconscious. Achievement of identity integration lends itself to the therapeutic indication for non-modified classical psychoanalytic technique.

4. In all cases, the interpretation of activated transference dispositions and the working through of their emotional implications in the context of technical neutrality characterize both psychoanalysis and truly psychoanalytic psychotherapies.

References

Bollas C: The Shadow of the Object: Psychoanalysis of the Unthought Known. New York, Columbia University Press, 1989

Caligor E, Kernberg OF, Clarkin JF, Yeomans FE: Psychodynamic Therapy for Personality Pathology: Treating Self and Interpersonal Functioning. Washington, DC, American Psychiatric Association Publishing, 2018

Coates S, Rosenthal J, Schecter D: September 11: Trauma and Human Bonds. New York, Routledge, 2003

Damasio A: Self Comes to Mind. New York, Vintage Books, 2010

Dammann G, Kernberg OF (eds): Schizoidie und schizoide Persönlichkeitsstörung, Stuttgart, Germany, Kohlhammer, 2019

Förstl H: Theory of Mind. Heidelberg, Germany, Springer, 2012

Freud S: Instincts and their vicissitudes (1915), in Standard Edition of the Complete Psychological Works of Sigmund Freud, Vol 14. Translated and edited by Strachey J. London, Hogarth, 1957, pp 111–116

Freud S: The ego and the id (1923), in Standard Edition of the Complete Psychological Works of Sigmund Freud, Vol 19. Translated and edited by Strachey J. London, Hogarth, 1961, pp 12–66

Green A: Le Travail du Négatif. Paris, Les Éditions de Minuit, 1993

Green A: Pourquoi les Pulsions de Destruction ou de Mort? Paris, Éditions du Panama, 2007

Hart S: Brain, Attachment, Personality. London, Karnac, 2008

Heim C, Nemeroff CB: The role of childhood trauma in the neurobiology of mood and anxiety disorders: preclinical and clinical studies. Biol Psychiatry 49(12):1023–1039, 2001

Isaacs S: The nature and function of phantasy. Int J Psychoanal 29:73–97, 1948

Jacobson E: The Self and the Object World. New York, International Universities Press, 1964

Kernberg OF: Object relations, affects, and drives. Psychoanal Inq 21(5):604–619, 2001

Kernberg OF: The concept of drive in the light of contemporary psychoanalytic theorizing, in Contemporary Controversies in Psychoanalytic Theory, Techniques, and Their Applications. New Haven, CT, Yale University Press, 2004a, pp 48–59

Kernberg OF: Hatred as a core affect of aggression, in Aggressivity, Narcissism, and Self-Destructiveness in the Psychoanalytic Process: New Developments in the Psychopathology and Psychotherapy of Severe Personality Disorders. New Haven, CT, Yale University Press, 2004b, pp 27–44

Kernberg OF: Psychoanalytic affect theory in the light of contemporary neurobiological findings. International Congress Series 1286:106–117, 2006

Kernberg OF: The concept of the death drive: a clinical perspective. Int J Psychoanal 90:1009–1023, 2009

Kernberg OF: The Inseparable Nature of Love and Aggression. Washington, DC, American Psychiatric Publishing, 2012

Kernberg OF: Resolution of Aggression and Recovery of Eroticism. Washington, DC, American Psychiatric Association Publishing, 2018

Klein M: Notes on some schizoid mechanisms. Int J Psychoanal 27:99–110, 1946

Krause R: Allgemeine Psychodynamische Behandlungs- und Krankheitslehre. Stuttgart, Germany, Kohlhammer, 2012

LeDoux J: The Deep History of Ourselves. New York, Viking, 2019

Northoff G: Neuropsychoanalysis in Practice. New York, Oxford University Press, 2011

Northoff G, Vatter J, Böker H: Das Selbst und das Gehirn, in Neuropsychodynamische Psychiatric. Edited by Böker H, Hartwich P, Northoff G. Berlin, Springer, 2016

Ogden TH: Reverie and Interpretation: Sensing Something Human. Northvale, NJ, Jason Aronson, 1997

Panksepp J: Affective Neuroscience: The Foundations of Human and Animal Emotions. New York, Oxford University Press, 1998

Panksepp J, Biven L: The Archaeology of Mind. New York, W.W. Norton, 2012

Rosenfeld HR: Notes on the psychopathology of confusional states in chronic schizophrenia. Int J Psychoanal 32:132–137, 1950

Roth G: Fühlen, Denken, Handeln wie das Gehirn Unser Verhalten Steuert. Frankfurt, Germany, Suhrkamp, 2001

Roth G, Dicke U: Funktionelle neuroanatomie des limbischen systems, in Neurobiologie Psychischer Störungen. Edited by Förstl J, Hautzinger M, Roth G. Berlin, Springer, 2006, pp 1–74

Roth G, Strüber N: Wie das Gehirn die Seele Macht. Stuttgart, Germany, Klett-Cotta, 2014

Solms M: The Feeling Brain. London, Karnac, 2015

Spillius EB, Milton J, Garvey P, et al: The New Dictionary of Kleinian Thought. London, Routledge, 2011

Stern D: The Interpersonal World of the Infant. New York, Basic Books, 1985

Svrakic DM, Divac-Jovanovic M: The Fragmented Personality. New York, Oxford University Press, 2019

Yeomans F, Clarkin JF, Kernberg OF: Transference Focused Psychotherapy for Borderline Personality Disorders: A Clinical Guide. Washington, DC, American Psychiatric Publishing, 2015

PART II

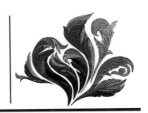

Technique

CHAPTER 3

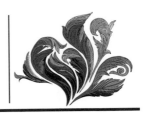

Extensions of Psychoanalytic Technique

THE MUTUAL INFLUENCES OF STANDARD PSYCHOANALYSIS AND TRANSFERENCE-FOCUSED PSYCHOTHERAPY

The objectives of this chapter include an effort to delimit more sharply the differences between "standard" psychoanalysis and transference-focused psychotherapy (TFP) and to review the particular difficulties that psychoanalytically and psychodynamically trained clinicians have in learning TFP. In delineating differences between standard psychoanalysis and TFP, I will discuss the contributions that recent developments in psychoanalytic technique offer to the optimal carrying out of TFP and present recent developments in TFP that may add significant contributions to "standard" psychoanalytic technique (Caligor and Stern 2021; Carsky 2021; Clarkin et al. 2021; Hersh 2021; Kernberg 2021; Yeomans et al. 2015).

Several questions arise immediately: First, can we really speak of "standard" psychoanalysis today, with alternative technical developments in contrasting schools and approaches to psychoanalytic treatment? Does the very term *standard* already imply an inappropriate restriction to the flexibility and richness of the psychoanalytic method that cannot be reduced to specific techniques? And, from a different perspective, is it *possible* to differentiate "standard" psychoanalysis clearly from the many variations of the model of applying psychoanalytic concepts that can be found in psychoanalytic psychotherapies? I hope to be able to respond to these questions in the course of what follows, and to be able to show that TFP is an important extension of psychoanalytic technique that permits the broadening of the application of psychoanalytic treatments to a severely ill segment of patients, those with severe personality disorders and the secondary symptoms of these disorders. These patients constitute a significant segment of the patient population we treat these days, and we currently utilize the application of specific modifications of psychoanalysis that clearly constitute an extension of psychoanalysis rather than a competing treatment approach. I shall propose that TFP, particularly in its recently extended form (TFP-E) as described by Eve Caligor and colleagues (2018; Caligor and Stern 2021), represents a fully developed, clearly formulated, and empirically validated form of psychoanalytic psychotherapy, representing the psychoanalytic psychotherapy closest to standard or classical psychoanalytic technique. TFP is potentially available to be integrated into an educational frame that prepares psychoanalysts to carry out alternative applications of the basic psychoanalytic method without confusion of these alternative applications, and with a clear enrichment of their respective indications, prognosis, and technique.

Differences Between Standard Psychoanalysis and Transference-Focused Psychotherapy

I have proposed in earlier work (Kernberg 2018) that the essential technical instruments that define the technique of psychoanalysis are the use of 1) free association as reflecting the basic task of the patient, as well as 2) interpretation, 3) transference analysis, 4) technical neutrality, and 5) countertransference as the fundamental technical instruments of the psychoanalyst. This simple classification may surprise, and, immediately, other aspects of psychoanalytic technique may emerge in the reader's mind: resistance, therapeutic alliance, containment, holding, character analysis, dream analysis, and so forth. I have proposed that all these other aspects of technique can be subsumed by the four basic ones that I defined as the analyst's tasks. I illustrate this with a few examples. For example, "resistance" reflects the activation of defensive mechanisms and constitutes part of what is analyzed by the method of interpretation, that consists, precisely, in the analysis of the unconscious conflict between impulse derivatives and defenses directed against them. "Containing" corresponds to the psychoanalyst's tolerance of the effects of the patient's projective identifications on the analyst's countertransference and the elaboration of the projected material as part of the utilization of countertransference analysis. The "therapeutic alliance," or alliance between the analyst in his or her role and the rational part of the patient's ego not involved in the present conflict explored in the transference, is strengthened by the analysis of the extent to which the patient's rational self or ego is dominated by defensive processes. The therapeutic alliance exists as a potential in healthier patients but may be essentially absent in very severe cases, and here the analytic task consists in the systematic analysis of negative transferences that, over time, permit the emergence and strengthening of the therapeutic alliance. The analysis of the transference permits the strengthening of the therapeutic alliance, in contrast to supportive psychotherapeutic techniques to strengthen the alliance by what may be called seductive reinforcement of positive transference developments. In short, and without entering into detailed exploration of all technical instruments, I believe that their systematic exploration brings us back to the four basic techniques of interpretation, transference analysis, technical neutrality, and countertransference utilization.

TFP is based on these same basic techniques: free association as the task of the patient and interpretation, transference analysis, technical neutrality, and countertransference utilization as the fundamental technical interventions of the psychotherapist. Each of these techniques, however, is employed with significant modification, so that a different picture evolves throughout time regarding the nature of the psychotherapeutic process. In what follows, I shall spell out these modifications and their consequences. In the process, both continuity and differentiation from standard analysis should become clear.

TFP is fully based on the fundamental principles of psychoanalytic technique with the core assumption that unconscious intrapsychic conflict is the dominant cause of personality disorders and their related and derived psychopathology. The systematic analysis of defensive operations and the direct emergence in consciousness of the corresponding

unconscious conflicts, particularly in the form of transference developments, permits the elaboration of these unconscious conflicts and their
resolution with enhanced ego strength and optimized psychological
functioning. By focusing on the treatment of the very severe forms of
personality disorders that mostly do not respond to standard psychoanalytic treatment, TFP has helped to highlight the predominance of
primitive defensive operation of these cases, the predominance of splitting mechanisms and related defenses in contrast to the predominance
of repression and related defenses at higher levels of psychopathology,
thus strengthening our experience in dealing with unconscious intrapsychic conflicts under such conditions.

INITIAL EVALUATION AND TREATMENT SETTING

The initial evaluation of patients, in theory, should be the same for better
and worse functioning patients, facilitating the differential diagnosis, indications for treatment, and assessing the prognosis of patients with personality disorders. A problematic practical tradition in psychoanalytic
education has been the tendency to neglect the careful diagnostic evaluation of patients, trusting in the diagnostic functions developing as part of
the very treatment. This corresponds to a parallel neglect of careful diagnostic evaluation as a result of a simplified, psychopharmacologically oriented trend in contemporary psychiatry. Psychiatric residents are trained
to focus exclusively on dominant symptoms and to neglect the analysis of
personality structure. All of this has combined in a regrettable lack of attention to careful diagnostic evaluation of all patients. I believe that TFP,
with its insistence on such careful early structural evaluation of the personality, has contributed significantly to the psychoanalytic field.

The method of working in each session, based on a combination of
the patient's instruction to carry out free association and the analyst or
therapist working with an "evenly suspended attention," even better,
"without memory or desire," is common to standard psychoanalytic
technique and TFP. It needs to be clarified that TFP is carried out in face-
to-face sessions and with a frequency of two or three sessions per week.
This differs, of course, from psychoanalytic treatment with use of the
couch and a frequency between three and five session per week. One
practical consequence of these arrangements is that, in standard psychoanalysis, the patients' free associations assume a much more important
function than the patients' nonverbal and general attitudinal expressions in the sessions. Psychoanalysis appropriately assumes that the
content of free associations, the communication of the patient's subjective experience by verbal communications will reflect a dominant way

to express the patient's internal life, while, in the case of severe psychopathology, the assumption is that unconscious conflicts and their derivatives will be expressed much more by nonverbal communications, both by the structure of the language itself and the general attitudinal expressions of the patient. In addition to the communicative function of the face-to-face approach, severe personality disorders are expressed quite early and dominantly by nonverbal behaviors, and the contribution of both features facilitates the diagnostic evaluation. One implication of this difference is that TFP has been able to focus on the patient's initial attitude and its transferential implications in a sharper way than what evolves in the treatment of less severe personality disorders. Here it is possible to differentiate what may be considered a "normal" object relationship established by behavior in the therapeutic encounter from the early transference distortions of that "normal" expected attitude.

Hans Loewald's (1960) characterization of the optimal psychoanalytic encounter is that of a patient who has problems, needs help, and expects the psychoanalyst to be honestly interested and knowledgeable and therefore to be of help. This patient is implicitly trusting the good intentions, knowledge, and experience of the psychoanalyst without attributing to the analyst omniscience nor omnipotence and is willing to explore his or her subjective life with the understanding that he or she may gain more understanding of it with the help of this analyst. In severe personality disorders, however, this theoretically expected optimal attitude of the patient is significantly absent or distorted from the very moment the treatment starts. The analyst, from the very first moment, is faced with more or less subtle or even dramatic manifestations of the distortion of this expected, normal attitude. TFP, in short, has the advantage of a potential rapid diagnosis of the nature of dominant transferences, not only because the more severe the psychopathology, the earlier and most powerfully transference developments distort the therapeutic interaction but also because the face-to-face encounter facilitates the early and precise diagnosis of the nature of these transference developments. It intensifies the standard psychoanalytic emphasis on the "total transference" (Joseph 1985, 2013).

INTERPRETATION

Interpretation in TFP follows the same principles and rules as interpretation in standard psychoanalysis: proceeding from surface to depth, from defense to impulse, the efforts to interpret at an optimal level of depth, and the selection of what is affectively dominant as indicating the highest priority of intervention, all are common principles that do not differentiate psychoanalysis from TFP. Differences emerge, however, in terms of the level of depth of interpretation. Severely affected personality disorders require a greater time and effort spent on the preliminary aspects of interpretive technique. This involves clarification of the content of the patient's communications and tactful confrontation with the patient's nonverbal manifestations that, together with the verbal content and the potentially intensive early activation of countertransference, determine the interpretive interventions. The combination of these features makes for a quantitative difference regarding the character of interpretive interventions in the two treatments.

TFP has contributed to the general method of interpretation with its stress on "affective dominance," a more specific expression of the Bionian focus on the "selected fact" (Yeomans et al. 2015). TFP proposes to use affective dominance as defined by the therapist on the basis of the combined analysis of the patient's verbal communication, nonverbal communication, and countertransference as the indicator for priority setting of interpretative intervention. This is a new contribution to general psychoanalytic technique but marks no difference between the two major technical approaches we are comparing. Also, the questions of what is surface and what is the depth, what is defense and what is impulse, become enriched by the treatment of pathology in which splitting mechanisms, projective identification, omnipotent control, and denial dominate. In contrast to cases where repression and its derivatives reflect the defensive structure and the interpretive focus is on the unknown repressed, in borderline cases the focus is on the affectively dissociated or split off, with frequent role reversals between what segment of the patient's experience is consciously invested and what is dissociatively denied although it continues in the patient's conscious awareness. Again, there is no basic difference here, but an expanded focus on what represents the surface and the deeper aspect of the material being explored: What is surface at one point may become what is split off and denied at another, with reversals of the role of these two aspects of the conflict.

TRANSFERENCE ANALYSIS

Transference analysis is systematically carried out in both standard psychoanalysis and TFP, with contemporary psychoanalytic object relations theory underlying both treatments. However, TFP highlights the fact that an entire dyadic unit of an internalized object relationship is expressed in the transference, which influences the scope of interpretive interventions. Practically, the projection onto the analyst of an internal object from the patient is complemented, often less visibly though, by the enactment, on the part of the patient, of the corresponding self-representation. The interpretative intervention has to cover both the analysis of the projection of the object and the parallel enactment of the correspondent self-representation. At other moments, a self-representation is projected onto the therapist while the patient enacts the representation of the corresponding object. The interpretation then has to cover the roles of both participants in the alternatively reverting activation of the same internalized, dissociated, or repressed internal relationship under the dominance of a corresponding positive or negative affect.

This technical approach is implicit in Kleinian interpretative interventions but has been made more explicit in the technical approach developed by TFP. From a broader perspective, it corresponds to development of the general psychoanalytic concept of the analysis of "the total transference" proposed by Betty Joseph (1985), which has been fundamentally influential in the development of the technique of TFP. Analysis of the total object relationship in the transference enriches transference interpretation.

In addition, the pervasive nature of acting out by patients with severe types of personality disorders is an important aspect of their life experiences during treatment. Our experience in carrying out TFP has indicated how often significant self-destructive acting out in the external environment may be so successfully dissociated from direct manifestations in the relationship with the therapist that it may not be diagnosed in time to prevent the patient from severe self-destructive effects in his life. We have learned to maintain an ongoing knowledge of the patient's external life to diagnose such successfully dissociated self-destructive behaviors and to bring them into the treatment situation. Sometimes, what becomes dominant in the countertransference of the therapist are reactions to the patient's "casual" mentioning of various events of his or her external life that, put together in the mind of the therapist, reflect an imminent danger to the patient's life or psychological survival of which the patient is unaware. For example, unacknowledged threats to the patient's employment, marriage, or financial health may be discovered first in the countertransference, on the basis of the therapist's monitoring of the patient's external life. At certain moments, denied external reality may create a countertransference anxiety that propels the subject into the realm of what is affectively dominant in the session and needs to be interpreted. As mentioned before, this awareness is a potential expansion of the analysis of the total transference, enriching the technical approach in this regard.

The approach to transference analysis summarized by David Tuckett (2005, 2019) points to two major phases of transference interpretation: The first consists of the expression of a predominant unconscious transference distortion with its attendant meaning. This is followed by a second phase in which the enactment of a significant internalized object relation from the past is explored. This approach corresponds to the TFP approach as well. However, severe personality disorders may experience severe regressions in the transference within which reality testing is lost, and the patient treats the present relationship with the therapist as if it were coincidental with the same relationship from the past. This patient no longer recognizes the difference between his or her activated unconscious fantasy and the actual reality of the interaction with the therapist. In other words, the activation of psychotic transference developments, or transference psychosis in a narrow sense, becomes a significant problem in the TFP of severe personality disorders (Kernberg 2019). At this point we have developed the technique of "incompatible realities," that is, the therapist's sharing with the patient his or her conviction that the patient's experience of the relationship or a specific aspect of it is unreal. The therapist would acknowledge the patient's conviction of what is going on while sharing his or her own, radically different conviction about it with the patient, thus acknowledging an incompatibility of their views without an attempt to resolve. Instead, the therapist invites the patient to jointly explore the nature of the issue regarding which they have such a totally divergent view and the significance of this issue as an expression of an important, deep conflict concerning the patient. In other words, the therapist's task becomes to define the psychotic nucleus activated in the transference as a precondition for jointly examining it without raising the question about its reality. This permits an elaboration of psychotic convictions as a profound reactivation of the unconscious past. The resolution of the corresponding conflict restores reality testing on the part of the patient together with his or her capacity to tolerate the corresponding conflict at a conscious, now realistic, level. I believe this is a significant contribution that TFP has made to psychoanalytic technique. It is perfectly compatible with standard psychoanalytic treatment as well, if the radical temporary deviation from technical neutrality that it implies can be tolerated by the analyst. This brings us to the next fundamental common technique and the differences in carrying it out, namely, technical neutrality.

TECHNICAL NEUTRALITY

Technical neutrality refers to the analyst not participating on one side of the unconscious conflict activated in the dominant transference. It represents, as Anna Freud (1936/1974) pointed out, a position of equal distance from the patient's id, superego, and acting ego and an involvement as an excluded "third other." This position implies a working relationship with the unconflicted part of the patient's ego, "the therapeutic alliance." Technical neutrality does not imply indifference but, rather, the therapist's concerned objectivity, the purpose of which is the full, unimpeded expression of the patient's transference. Here TFP has developed a technical modification significantly different from a standard psychoanalytic approach, namely, the temporary suspension of technical neutrality in order to protect the treatment frame, the life and survival of the patient and others involved with the patient, under circumstances of severe acting out that threatens the treatment. In such instances, the therapist takes measures to establish conditions that assure the patient's maintaining ordinary social behavior consistent with the therapeutic arrangements. Practically, abandonment of technical neutrality is indicated in the face of dangerous acting out, severe self-mutilating behavior, suicidal attempts, dangerous antisocial behavior, or severe infringement of the rights, safety, or health of others, including the therapist. Departure from technical neutrality may be indicated to establish (or reestablish) the conditions necessary for the continuation of the treatment under conditions of acting out dangerous or destructive behavior that cannot be managed by interpretative means. If the behavior is not amenable to clarification and interpretation, limits must be established as a condition for continuing the treatment, which clearly represents an abandonment of technical neutrality. When such intervention becomes necessary, the therapist continues the interpretation of the corresponding unconscious conflict while maintaining the corresponding restrictions on the patient's behavior, to be followed by the analysis of the reasons for which the patient necessitated such a modification in the treatment. Thus, eventually, the interpretation of the function and meaning of this episode restores technical neutrality at the end of this process. This clearly constitutes a required and effective modification of standard psychoanalytic treatment in the treatment of very severe personality disorders.

Technical neutrality also involves a more subtle aspect of the formulation of interpretive interventions, as implied in Fred Busch's (2014) excellent comments on psychoanalytic technique. The analyst should not raise questions that implicitly indicate the analyst's preference for certain behaviors of the patient or put into question certain aspects of the patient behavior, and indicate, in short, the emergence of the analyst's "desire." Attention to the patient's external reality may reveal behaviors that imply a clear denial of reality aspects of the patient's external life. This denial in turn facilitates the severe acting out of self-destructive behavior and becomes part of what is left out from verbal communication in the transference. The denial of reality may emerge as a certain confusion or lack of clarity in the patient's communications. In TFP, the task of the therapist is, first, to clarify what seems incomprehensible or strange and, second, to explore to what extent the patient is able to carry out an objective assessment of it. On the surface, the therapist, raising a series of questions about what is really going on that cannot be understood, appears to be acting outside of technical neutrality when what he or she is attempting to do is to interpret the patient's denial of aspects of reality. The active efforts in this regard may differentiate TFP from the traditional, major effort in standard psychoanalysis not to raise questions in order to protect technical neutrality. It is a technique that may well be integrated into standard psychoanalytic work if and when such complications evolve in the treatment of a patient in analysis.

Countertransference Utilization

It is well known that the intensity of countertransference reactions, the fast and rapidly changing affective impact on the analyst's emotional experience in the sessions, is particularly marked in the treatment of severe personality disorders. Rapid development of intense transference regression and sudden shifts in the transference may produce countertransference reactions as early alerting signals in the analyst of what is emerging in the patient's communications. In TFP, therefore, a focused alertness to countertransference reactions is a constant aspect of the therapist's work and at times significantly influences the decision-making process of the therapist about what is affectively dominant in the transference. In both psychoanalysis and TFP, the task for the therapist is to tolerate the development of the countertransference experience. This permits its full intrapsychic development as part of the effort to clarify the meaning of the countertransference reaction and to elucidate to what extent the meaning of that reaction derives from the patient's or from the analyst's corresponding conflicts, including the extent to which this countertransference reaction permits further clarification of what is developing in the transference. What has been learned in this complex and fast intrapsychic process of the therapist ends up as the possibility of an enriched interpretation of transference meanings. Thus, countertransference is not communicated directly to the patient but is used as an important element in the construction of transference interpretation. If countertransference is excessive, cannot be controlled, and is somehow expressed, even if only partially, in the therapist's reaction toward the patient, it has to be acknowledged as an issue that the therapist has introduced into the treatment, and not denied. If the patient confronts the therapist with this countertransference acting out, and this happens to be a realistic observation, it has to be accepted, but without leading the analyst to share with the patient the unconscious motivations of his or her own behavior. These general principles operate in standard psychoanalysis as well as in psychoanalytic psychotherapy. However, in some psychoanalytic orientations, particularly among psychoanalysts with a relational approach, direct communication to the patient of the countertransference may be incorporated as part of their psychoanalytic technique. The only potential problem, in the case of the treatment of very severe personality disorders, is that countertransference reactions may acquire very primitive aggressive, dependent, or sexual aspects that are frightening or difficult to tolerate for the therapist, a specific task in the learning of TFP.

By the same token, when the TFP therapist comes to terms with the activation of primitive, regressive fantasies in the countertransference and dares to experience them fully without feeling threatened by them, he or she also becomes freer to interpret the corresponding transferences being expressed by the patient during the sessions. The therapist tends to become freer to explore primitive forms of sadomasochistic, perverse, envious, revengeful, and aggressively dependent behavior directly in the transference that initially might have led the therapist to assume that the patient would not be able to tolerate that depth of this experience. We have discovered with very ill patients, if the therapist tolerates talking about the patient's primitive wishes and fears directly in the hours, thus providing a cognitive frame, the patient, in turn, can tolerate them much better than the therapist feared. This may be an important emotionally corrective experience for the therapist. Experienced TFP psychotherapists may become more relaxed in interpreting particularly primitive, aggressive, and sexual fantasies of their patients, within an appropriate cognitive frame that provides a holding structure to previously feared primitive fears and desires.

In summary, TFP really does not differ in the basic utilization of the fundamental four techniques characterizing psychoanalytic treatment. There are some differences that emerge in the application of these basic techniques, such as in dream analysis. Free associations to segments of manifest dream content are a problematic task in the early stages of treatment with TFP. The capacity for carrying out free association is slower in TFP than in patients with an indication for standard psychoanalytic treatment. I believe this and other examples, however, don't change the basic correspondence between TFP and psychoanalysis, with quantitative differences in the application of the various aspects of these basic techniques that have been outlined. There emerges an overall different quality to the two treatments when observed over a period of time, except regarding the frequency of sessions and the face-to-face contact between patient and therapist in TFP. The specific modifications of TFP allow expansion of psychoanalytic treatment to those most severe cases that would not seem likely to respond to standard psychoanalytic treatment and thus extends the reach of psychoanalysis.

Training Issues: Controversies and Experience

I shall discuss ways of working as a TFP therapist that may relate to earlier training experiences and identity and how TFP therapists approach their therapeutic work. In terms of the impact of prior training experiences, there are advantages and disadvantages of training in standard psychoanalysis followed by training in TFP, training in TFP preceded by general training in various modes of psychoanalytic psychotherapies that combine expressive and supportive techniques, training without previous or parallel psychoanalytic training, and training in TFP for therapists who have not had any training in psychoanalytic psychotherapy of any kind. Our group at Cornell is invested in research on process and outcome of TFP and is made up mostly by psychotherapists who have had many years of "standard" psychoanalytic experience. All of us also have had many years of general psychoanalytic psychotherapy experience and are deeply interested in psychoanalytic theory, psychoanalytic technique, and how they apply to psychotherapeutic theory and technique. Because of our experiences with therapists and psychoanalysts we are training locally as well as in various European, North American, and Latin American countries, and in China, we have been able to observe specific problems in training and specific difficulties that therapists have in relation to their professional background, and we have developed some general understanding of related training problems that I will examine here. This is not a comprehensive approach covering all possible difficulties and developments but reflects frequent experiences that we have found to be helpful in our teaching, supervision, and in conducting both psychoanalysis and TFP. I have organized these observations in terms of the various aspects of technique that have been summarized above, both their effective and problematic employment according to therapists' different background and training.

DIAGNOSIS AND GOALS

As mentioned above, diagnostic evaluation is unfortunately inadequate at all levels of psychoanalytic training institutes, with strong biases even against carrying out a careful initial evaluation being quite prevalent. This failure is often rationalized as a fear that careful diagnostic evaluation may deter patients from entering treatment or may alter the nature of the transference. I believe these fears are totally unfounded. Ideological positions critical of "medical diagnosis," disappointment in and distrust of classical psychiatry, therapists' resentment of the superficiality of the descriptive classifications in contemporary psychiatric settings, lack of adequate clinical training of therapists who enter psychoanalytic or psychotherapeutic training without having a psychiatric or clinical psychological or clinical social work background, and lack of personal clinical experience in a general psychiatric service as part of a therapist's overall clinical training are all issues that combine in this lack of diagnostic skill and practice. I can only stress the enormous value of an initial diagnosis in terms of the *structure* of the personality, the diagnosis of the predominant nature of the defensive organization, and the severity of the compromise of identity and object relations and its importance in the decision of whether psychoanalysis or psychoanalytic psychotherapy, particularly TFP, is the optimal choice of treatment.

A simple and fundamental set of questions that can be answered in the course of such a careful evaluation is: What are the main objectives the patient brings to the treatment—what does he or she want to change or achieve? And what are the main objectives of the therapist—what does he or she want to change or achieve? In general, it seems essential that even if they have several divergent objectives for the treatment, patient and therapist coincide in at least one basic issue that the treatment is geared to change or resolve. This may seem almost trivial, but it becomes directly and fundamentally relevant at points of intense negative transference, when the patient's very continuation of the treatment comes into question. But the most important result of a good diagnostic evaluation is the appropriate indication for a modality of psychoanalytic treatment, with implicit prognostic implications: It reflects the expanding realm of psychodynamic treatments for multiple types and severities of psychological illness.

VERBAL COMMUNICATION AND FREE ASSOCIATION

Here the advantages of standard psychoanalytic training for the TFP therapist appear very clearly: In all psychoanalytic orientations, the emphasis on free association as the patient's task appears to be important and is reflected in the analyst's careful attention to the patient's verbal communication, the tolerance of prolonged silences, and the attention to the manifestation of defensive operations revealed in the distortion of verbal communications. Therapists without psychoanalytic training are more prone to neglect the importance of this aspect of the patient's contribution to the work in the sessions and are more easily tempted to be seduced into an ongoing dialogue with the patient that then serves to express defensive operations that are more difficult to diagnose and analyze. This constitutes a particular difficulty, then, for TFP therapists who do not have that background in their learning experiences.

Another related problem has to do with a systematic distortion of language, the patient's talking in either totally disjointed ways that don't permit the deepening of any particular subject or the typical rapid dissociative shift from one subject to another that creates chaos in verbal communication. This is a frequent problem in severe personality disorders that usually goes hand in hand with parallel distortions in the patient's nonverbal behavior, leading to failure to attend to the total problem and its eventual analytic exploration. In that regard, psychoanalysts trained to be very attentive to free association may be seduced for extended periods of time to tolerate a patient's relatively abstract language that permits the patient to avoid concrete emotional experiences with others. TFP is so intensively involved in assessing the momentary dominant object relationship in the transference that this misuse of language can be rapidly diagnosed.

This close attention to the verbal material also permits rapid diagnosis of the narcissistic use of language to compete with the therapist, the patient acting as his or her own supervisor and as supervisor of the therapist's interventions, that emerges more quickly in the treatment of narcissistic personalities in TFP. Therapists with experience in TFP may be able to diagnose the misuse of free association in the case of narcissistic pathology by the patient's attitude of continuing to "free associate" while ignoring concrete interventions of the therapist, so that an attitude of depreciation and dismissal of what the therapist is saying may become clearly evident earlier than when the patient is associating on the couch.

Because defensive confusion about reality situations in the patient's communications may gradually emerge over the sessions in the course of psychoanalysis, and the frequency of sessions provides the analyst an experience of the same confusing problem repeated over an extended period of time, this may gradually lead to its interpretative resolution. Thus, defensive confusion may eventually be resolved in the course of the treatment, at the cost of an extended period of time in which it remains masked. That time element protects technical neutrality but may also obscure subtle acting out carried out before the analyst has a clear sense of what is going on in the patient's external life. In contrast, the intensity of transference developments in severe psychopathology and the heightened alertness of the TFP therapist to what is going on in the patient's external life may facilitate the therapist investigating and intervening more rapidly in resolving the obscure nature of the patient's communications, accelerating the diagnosis and treatment, and protecting the patient. But at times this carries the risk of loss of technical neutrality in the process. However, the alertness to this very use of linguistic communication to obscure a significant problem in external reality is something highlighted in TFP. The lower frequency of sessions and the urgency of intervening under conditions of severe acting out require an active interpretative engagement that accelerates the rhythm of treatment with severe psychopathology, helpful in those cases, while, with healthier patients, the intensity of inquiring may foster acting out of the countertransference. Different speeds and intensity of interpretive work are required by different severities of psychopathology and regression.

INTERVENTIONS

As mentioned previously, the severity of acting out, the rapidity of sudden changes, given the predominance of splitting mechanisms, may require rapid interventions. TFP therapists may have to limit themselves to clarification and confrontation before there is sufficient clarity of the transference meanings to interpret in depth. However, the TFP therapist's closeness to patients' primitive affective developments trains the therapist to verbalize such conflicts and be prepared earlier to interpret them in depth. Well-trained TFP therapists may be less afraid to spell out primitive transferences directly, particularly involving intense aggression, without fear of the patient's reacting in a counteraggressive way and may be more prepared to analyze the patient's reactions to their interpretations. Psychoanalysts may be more reluctant, as mentioned before, to directly interpret primitive aggression in the transference.

In both modalities, certain transference developments are first and predominantly acted out with third parties, and it becomes a technical question to what extent they should be interpreted directly in the transference. In standard psychoanalysis, with less intense transferences, it may take some time to bring conflictual aspects of the relationship between patient and analyst into the transference if the patient's focus is predominantly on what is going on in the relationship between the patient and an outside party. In TFP, the process is facilitated enormously by more intense and negative transferences, so that the therapist's attempts to analyze the unconscious meanings of a conflict with a third party tend to actuate the conflictual relationship between patient and therapist and facilitate analysis of the transference. Transferences are more pronounced and volatile with the severe personality disorders, making their presence known from the beginning of treatment and providing the analyst numerous opportunities to interpret their meaning to the patient.

In short, the rapid development of affectively dominant transferences in TFP facilitates transference interpretation and accelerates the entire interpretive process. An open question that remains is to what extent some of these findings may be applied to a more rapid intervention, from the position of technical neutrality of the analyst, in a standard psychoanalytic treatment.

One difficulty for therapists without standard psychoanalytic training is the natural way of organizing interpretations in terms of focusing on the defensive aspect of the conflict first, then on the motivation of this defense, before spelling out what the patient is defending against and what activated the corresponding impulse. This natural ordering between defense, motive, and impulse is a very important structural element of interpretation, often almost unconsciously attended to in the supervision of psychoanalytic treatment carried out by psychoanalytic candidates. With neurotic-level patients, this is the proper ordering of interpretation, given the predominance of repression as defense against unwanted/intolerable affects. However, the defensive structure found in personality disorders centers around splitting and projective mechanisms; therefore, interpretations of defense, motive, and impulse are geared more toward integration of dissociated dyadic units of self and other rather than of repressed experience. TFP excels in the analysis of a defensive dyadic—self and object—structured transference development directed against a temporary opposite dyadic unit now representing the impulsive side of the conflict.

Because the attitude of the patient in face-to-face treatment of severe personality disorders so quickly reveals the transferential distortion of the assumed "normal" patient attitude, it is easier for the TFP psychotherapist to quickly recognize the nature of transference expression and acting out so that a faster and greater early awareness of it coincides with the challenge of formulating transference interpretations in ways that are acceptable to the patient.

Here the combined training in standard psychoanalysis and TFP has an enormous advantage. This advantage has only been recognized in recent times, in the few psychoanalytic institutes in which training in TFP is part of the general educational analytic program. I believe it should become a standard aspect of psychoanalytic training to train candidates in TFP as well. The fear has been widespread that such training in psychoanalytic psychotherapy would "dilute" the training in psychoanalytic technique. In our experience, to the contrary, spelling out clearly a theory of psychoanalytic technique as it applies to standard psychoanalysis, in contrast to its modifications in psychoanalytic psychotherapies, helps the therapist to shift approaches easily between these two related, yet clearly differentiated, ways of operating, enriching therapists' technical skills and freedom rather than creating the risk of confusion. In this regard, the coincidence of the underlying theory of psychoanalysis and TFP is an important theoretical basis that facilitates the alternative use of these two modalities of treatment according to their optimal indicators in each individual case.

Therapists learning TFP who have had training in mentalization-based therapy (MBT) find the diagnostic evaluation of a predominant dyadic relation in the transference a very comfortable approach. MBT focuses sharply on the patient's distorted experiences of the therapist's intention and behavior, with the intention of improving the patient's realistic perception of the therapist and his or her own distortions of it. This is also the first step in TFP's evaluation of the nature of the presently prominent dyad. What the MBT therapist has to learn is the dyadic nature of the patient's perception of the other related to the perception of self, not in order to normalize it but to prepare for the interpretation of the interchange of self and object identification in the transference.

The MBT approach may be considered as coincidental with the initial stage of transference interpretation in TFP.

In our experience, treatment of severe personality disorders with TFP not only permits analysis of severe regressive transferences from the very beginning of treatment but also recognizes that older biases regarding the "fragility" of very ill patients and their "hypersensitivity" to any interpretation of the transference, or even to any interpretive intervention, are in error. We have found that patients are surprisingly able to understand and work with interpretations from early on in the treatment.

When interpretations are formulated in clear and simple ways, starting from the surface, that is, the patient's conscious perceptions and behavior, and gradually deepen their communication of the total object relationship involved in the patient's reactions, even complex transference developments may be interpretively clarified. This has been observed even with patients in intense affective crisis or severe emotional withdrawal—some schizoid patients, or patients with a history of extremely traumatic experiences.

Some patients create an atmosphere of such fragility and incapacity to tolerate a direct approach that therapists may become particularly cautious in their treatment. In standard psychoanalytic treatment such difficulties may emerge in the form of long-standing silences and lack of verbal response to the analyst's interventions, and present additional difficulties to interpret the corresponding transference because of the limited manifestations of nonverbal aspects of the patient's behavior and correspondent countertransference fears of "retraumatizing" the patient. This can result in an unconscious collusion with the patient to avoid discussing any material that is affectively laden or challenging to the patient, resulting in a stalled treatment. In TFP the nonverbal behavior that accompanies such apparent closure of the channel of verbal communication as an expression of an unbearable closeness to the memory of very traumatic experiences may more easily be interpreted in the light of the present dyadic situation thus generated: the activation of the experience of an intensely sadistic authority that considers any expression of negative feelings as forbidden, dangerous, highly traumatic, and "punishable."

The analysis of the corresponding transference that emerges in the total expression of the patient's behavior in relation to the therapist permits resolution of these apparent stalemates, such as endless periods of silence or silent protests, much more rapidly than happens in the psychoanalysis of these types of patients. This apparent blocking of communication in the treatment situation as an expression of a specific transference development was observed by Edith Jacobson (1971) in the treatment of severe depression. She discovered that, under conditions when patients were practically dedicating all their efforts in the session to demonstrate to the analyst the analyst's incompetence in helping them, and the sense they conveyed that they were content that they themselves were condemned to internal suffering, these developments reflected the identification of the patient with a sadistic superego that condemned themselves to suffer. Simultaneously, the corresponding projection of this attack and of the experience of an oppressed self onto the therapist permitted the patient unconsciously to enact the dominant destructive aspect of that identification.

In more general terms, the activation of very primitive transferences may express deep conflicts that have never been experienced in a cognitive symbolized language by the patient but are only "remembered" as a disposition to very early behavioral interactions. We do now know that severe traumatization in the first 2 years of life may not be set down in cognitive memory leading to reactivated memory of such experiences, because emotional cognition of these early experiences is erased because of the immaturity of the hippocampus and the correspondent lack of development of explicit long-term memory. The earliest traumatic experiences are fixated in the distortion of early behavior patterns under the impact of such experiences that cannot be remembered. They only show up as reactivation of emotional responses that can be emotionally understood as reactivated object relations without being able to lead to correspondent categorical memories and have to be interpreted in their present transferential functions alone (Braten 2011). The analysis of extended silences and of chronic anxiety states in schizoid personalities with very little accompanying intrapsychic fantasy life may be worked through in the systematic analysis of the dominant object relations in the transference, particularly the role reversal between a persecutory object and its victim. The utilization of countertransference analysis becomes a fundamental instrument under such conditions, with careful attention of the extent to which one's interpretive intervention modifies the situation that is being explored, always maintaining an appropriate openness to alternative meanings of newly evolving situations.

TRANSFERENCE INTERPRETATION

The analysis of projective identifications activated in the transference that places the therapist into the role of the projected object representation goes hand-in-hand with the enactment by the patient of the corresponding self-representation, or, to the contrary, the projection of the patient's self-representation of the dissociated internalized object relationship onto the therapist, while the patient identifies with the corresponding object representation. TFP is specifically focused on the activation of such dyadic units and their ultimate development into triadic units when the therapist, an "excluded outside third element" interpretively threatens the activated dyadic relationship in some specific way.

Interpreting transference in TFP tends to bring about rapid shifts in the nature of the transference, even if temporary ones, with frequent reversal to the original transference situation that had been interpreted. For example, the patients may interpret the behavior of the therapist as an attack that clearly reflected a past experience with a significant parental object. This may reemerge repeatedly under different circumstances and may be analyzed and apparently resolved, only to return at some point. However, the working through of the issue shows in the gradual decrease of the intensity of the pattern and in the developing capacity of the patient to integrate the mutually split idealized and persecutory relation to the same object. When this development does not take place, it indicates that this relationship serves defensive purposes against an underlying, different relation that needs to be analyzed. These sequences emerge more quickly in TFP than in standard psychoanalysis because of the ongoing focus on the dominant dyadic relationship, the rapid impact of the interpretive interventions, which facilitates transference analysis but also highlights cases where that is not effective. In TFP, the question is what is the patient doing with the interpretive work in between the sessions and to what extent is the transference work affecting the patient's external life as well as his or her developments in the sessions. These developments usually happen at a much slower pace in standard psychoanalysis, where the lack of effectiveness of therapeutic interventions emerges more slowly. In this regard, the experiences in TFP should influence standard psychoanalytic work, potentially accelerating the focus on working through of the transference interpretation with attention to time utilization. Psychoanalytic training focuses on patients developing gradual insight into conflictual issues in the course of the sessions, while TFP focuses on relatively fast diagnostic assessment of conflicts and related therapeutic interventions.

The question can be raised, however, to what extent frequent therapeutic interventions, and the acceleration of an interpretive process, might foster an abandonment of technical neutrality and do injustice to the necessary time for intrapsychic elaboration and change. André Green (2012) pointed out that, because of the splitting operations and the rapid shift from one dominant transference situation into the next, with consequent lack of deepening, rapid interventions are required in patients with severe personality disorders. These interventions should take into consideration this change from one transference disposition to the next while, at the same time, focusing on the avoidance of in-depth experiencing as a common element to all these various shifts.

TFP training directs the therapist to be "impatient" in any particular session, in terms of utilizing time maximally, while being very patient in terms of the long-term nature that working through deep-seated problems requires. Some of this spirit might be helpful to avoid the defense of "slowing down" the analytic process on the part of many patients, particularly those with secondary gain of illness and, of course, as an expression of patients' effective defensive operations. This problem brings us back to the "phobic reaction" that patients with severe, concrete traumatic experiences in the past may induce in their analyst or therapist, patients who actively refuse to discuss their past traumatic experiences or convey the message that such a discussion would be highly traumatic for them.

I believe that this is a quite prevalent fantasy within the psychoanalytic psychotherapy environment and reflects the fear of confronting the negative transference implications hidden behind such prohibitive behavior on the part of patients. TFP has acquired experience in carrying out systematic analyses of why patients are afraid to deal with certain issues of their past and what that fear implies in terms of transference development, thus approaching the analysis of traumatic situations without fear of "retraumatizing" patients. In our experience, this fear seems unfounded. When the patient's reluctance to explore certain material is approached from the analysis of the transference implications of such reluctance, the patient feels safer to eventually discuss the underlying trauma. It is almost as if the "retraumatization" lies in the therapist's collusion with the patient's belief that certain material must remain sequestered and cannot be discussed. Both tacitly agree that certain topics are forbidden and collude to leave painful past experiences unaddressed. Our approach may be of help if incorporated into the conduct of standard psychoanalytic technique. Needless to say, tact and timing are important.

TECHNICAL NEUTRALITY, COMMON SENSE, AND ORDINARY LIFE

Here, there is a clear technical modification that TFP has introduced for the treatment of patients who, under ordinary psychoanalytic treatment arrangements, would break up the therapeutic relationship because of dangerous uncontrolled acting out or dangerous developments in the patient's condition or life situation that would interfere with the continuation of the treatment. Technical neutrality is reinstated analytically in TFP once the issue that motivated the deviation from technical neutrality has been resolved, and it protects the treatment from shifting into a supportive modality. It protects, in short, the essential analytic nature of the treatment.

Technical neutrality, however, also may be threatened by the increased "activity" of the analyst who interprets transference developments relatively rapidly and frequently. There is a danger that the analyst's value systems, his or her particular approach to reality, may unduly influence the patient, such as in raising questions regarding aspects of reality that are not clear, and where significant acting out may apparently occur outside the material expressed in the hours, even with an approach of "total transference" analysis. This is an important issue that may acquire truly existential implications.

I believe that there are some basic aspects of ordinary life that the patient must work through to lead a less impoverished life. I am referring to the requirements of the three basic spheres of activity, in work and profession, love and sex, social life and creativity. It seems reasonable to expect the patient to have some kind of gratifying functioning in these three major areas of life and that patients with severe restrictions in them warrant help and treatment. Practically, this implies a "common sense" evaluation on the part of the therapist of how the patient is functioning in his or her total life. Such assessment begins with the initial diagnostic evaluation and should continue throughout the treatment. It is important, in this regard, that the therapist use common sense in deciding what, given this patient's life situation, background, education, capacity, social environment, and so forth, would be available to the patient if the patient were not imprisoned in this illness. We help the patient become aware of these issues and explore with the patient what can be changed in those areas of failure or inhibition. It may be unavoidable that the analyst's value systems enter this picture. In this regard, an implicit question about the maintenance of technical neutrality is true enough—particularly with very ill patients. On the other side of this alternative is the analyst's potential blindness to significant life limitations that the patient unconsciously is trying to maintain by attempting to "brainwash" the analyst or therapist into accepting that "that's the limit of what the patient can do." It seems important that the analyst and the patient explore in themselves to what extent objective common sense warrants intervention in some areas, or to what extent there is a risk of a *furor sanandi*, that is, a therapist's excessive investment in creating an ideal life for the patient, which may be affecting technical neutrality and the treatment. This is an issue to be explored in psychoanalysis as well as in TFP, and it sometimes is not explored in analysis because of the relative slowness with which things develop, and where less urgency regarding major life decisions provides more time for reflection. With borderline patients, their active, self-destructive behavior threatens their survival and forces a faster way of dealing with these issues in TFP.

Of the three main domains of life mentioned above, engagement in love and sex are usually the last to improve. After all, to some extent all patients, except a very privileged minority, have to work and develop their interactions with others as an important part of social survival, while the inhibition of love life may lead to severe loneliness but is less crucial to overall survival. At the same time, there are so many social biases, inhibitions, and limitations to the achievement of a full and gratifying love life that it is important to recognize that psychoanalysis has been of crucial importance in pointing to the infantile inhibition of normal development of this area of life and the importance of exploring it in great detail as a universal human problem. In practice, this is a dimension that tends to be neglected throughout the entire realm of psychoanalytic psychotherapies, and even in psychoanalysis itself.

It seems reasonable to affirm that, while concrete sexual problems may often be resolved with cognitive behavioral interventions, the capacity to love and to integrate love and erotism is an area where psychoanalytic psychotherapies, including standard psychoanalysis, fulfill an essential therapeutic role, and therefore it is a part of the responsibility of the therapist to deal with this issue. In the course of psychoanalytic treatment, patients' difficulties in their love life typically emerge in great detail, but the very personal aspects of their sexual functioning may be successfully kept from being examined in the transference, even in the hands of very experienced psychoanalysts from all orientations. TFP is faced with the more dramatic and severe incapacities to be involved in a satisfactory love relationship. This emerges as a major problem for many patients and, therefore, has been at the center of our therapeutic work. The analysis of severely regressive sadomasochistic sexual developments and the oedipal and preoedipal conflicts that inhibit a patient's establishing a satisfactory love relationship with a significant other are essential concerns for both TFP and psychoanalysis. Here, the urgency of intervention in severely disturbed love relations affects TFP more than in standard psychoanalysis where, in general, conflicts in the area of love relations emerge more slowly and gradually and offer more time for understanding and resolution. This topic requires specific attention in the training of therapists in carrying out TFP. Technical neutrality, in short, is equally important and carried out in psychoanalysis and in TFP, with the temporary limitations in TFP referred to above. But it may be at higher risk of being challenged in TFP, and TFP therapists with training in psychoanalytic institutes have a higher level of therapeutic experience in this regard.

COUNTERTRANSFERENCE AND PRIOR TRAINING

Here again, psychoanalytic training, or rather, the experience of a personal psychoanalysis, is a very helpful precondition for optimal TFP training. We have found that the experience in a personal, high-quality psychoanalytic psychotherapy may also serve this function. The intensity of countertransference reactions induced by the regressive transferences of severe personality disorders becomes an evident, dominant issue in the training of TFP therapists. The task of disentangling the aspects of this countertransference reflecting the reasonable reactions to the transference from the activation of specific unconscious conflicts of the therapist in the therapeutic interaction, an essential aspect of countertransference analysis, is strongly supported by the therapist's personal psychotherapeutic experience as a patient. Therapists without that experience are more seriously exposed to countertransference acting out and the correspondent loss of the position of technical neutrality.

But the very intensity and primitivity of transference regression of borderline personality organization patients in TFP may facilitate the therapist's direct contact with primitive aggressive and sadomasochistic sexual and self-destructive impulses and deepen their psychoanalytic understanding by the therapist. This speaks for the advantages of TFP training as part of psychoanalytic training. Essentially, the technique of countertransference utilization in TFP is not different from the correspondent technique in psychoanalytic training. As mentioned before, TFP, in this regard, coincides with the technical approach of contemporary Kleinian, ego psychological, and French approaches and is different from the relational approach that includes selected communications of the countertransference.

It needs to be acknowledged that some TFP students who have never had a psychotherapeutic experience as a patient evince a surprisingly open and reflective awareness of deep emotional experiences and conflicts in themselves, which facilitates their training, in contrast to the serious learning difficulties that most psychodynamically naïve trainees usually present. But it also needs to be recognized that some trained psychoanalysts may present characterological difficulties that limit their countertransference exploration and understanding.

Conclusion

TFP is an extension and modification of standard psychoanalysis based on the utilization of the same essential psychoanalytic techniques, but with quantitative modifications geared to the treatment of the most severe segment of personality disorders, which tend to not be treatable by standard analysis proper. The development of this treatment and experiences in carrying it out have led to the discovery of new technical approaches and attitudes that may support and enrich standard psychoanalytic treatment, while, at the same time, affirming the importance of psychoanalytic training for psychoanalytic psychotherapy. Therapists who are trained in general psychoanalytic psychotherapies but not in psychoanalysis may manifest specific difficulties and potential limitations in their work. TFP includes some features, such as the importance of free association and the organization of interpretations in terms of the analysis of defense, motivation, and impulse, that are facilitated by psychoanalytic education, while, on the other hand, the discovery of the helpfulness of modification of technical neutrality under certain circumstances, the analysis of "incompatible realities," and the acceleration of interventions under conditions of severe acting out represent illustrations of how TFP enriches standard psychoanalytic treatment.

The most general recommendation emerging from this comparative study is the great advantage in a systematic training in TFP within psychoanalytic institutes as a true enrichment of technical training, and the general advantage of psychoanalysis as a profession to be considered as a broad spectrum of treatment approaches based upon the combined utilization of psychoanalytic techniques, with specific modifications to be organized in specific forms of psychoanalytic psychotherapy. I am suggesting that TFP may be the closest modification to standard psychoanalysis proper, but there are other derived approaches that deserve to be explored. For example, Eve Caligor and colleagues (2018, 2021) have proposed the extension of TFP (TFP-E) to personality disorders that are less severe, where the lack of sufficient severity and the limitation of their symptomatology indicate that such a modified treatment approach may be optimal.

In short, I believe that TFP is a legitimate extension of psychoanalysis proper, in contrast to the traditional attitude within psychoanalytic institutes that consider psychoanalytic psychotherapy as "diluted" psychoanalysis. In contrast to rejecting "standard" psychoanalytic technique, while no clear generally accepted definition of standard psychoanalytic technique has ever emerged, one of the important contributions of TFP has been the effort to clearly define and manualize this approach. This has permitted empirical research that has already demonstrated the effectiveness of TFP and challenges standard psychoanalysis to be equally defined, manualized, and empirically investigated. The beginning of this process may already have started but needs to be accelerated in a world around us that in turn is rapidly changing.

References

Braten S: Intersubjektive partizipation: bewegungen des virtuellen anderen bei säuglingen und erwaøchsenen. Psyche 65:832–861, 2011

Busch F: Creating a Psychoanalytic Mind. London, Routledge, 2014

Caligor E, Stern B: Editorial introduction to the special issue: recent advances in transference-focused psychotherapy: extending and refining the treatment model. Psychodyn Psychiatry 49(2):173–177, 2021

Caligor E, Kernberg OF, Clarkin JF, Yeomans FE: Psychodynamic Therapy for Personality Pathology: Treating Self and Interpersonal Functioning. Washington, DC, American Psychiatric Association Publishing, 2018

Carsky M: Managing countertransference in the treatment of personality disorders. Psychodyn Psychiatry 49(2):339–360, 2021

Clarkin JF, Caligor E, Sowislo J: TFP extended: development and recent advances. Psychodyn Psychiatry 49(2):188–214, 2021

Freud A: The ego and the mechanisms of defense, in The Writings of Anna Freud, Vol 2. New York, International Universities Press, 1974, pp 3–176

Green A: La Clinique Psychoanalytique Contemporaire. Paris, Les Éditions d' Ithaque, 2012

Hersh RG: Applied transference-focused psychotherapy: an overview and update. Psychodyn Psychiatry 49(2):273–295, 2021

Jacobson E: Depression: Comparative Studies of Normal, Neurotic, and Psychotic Conditions. New York, International Universities Press, 1971

Joseph B: Transference: the total situation. Int J Psychoanal 66:447–454, 1985

Joseph B: Here and now: my perspective. Int J Psychoanal 94:1–5, 2013

Kernberg OF: Resolution of Aggression and Recovery of Eroticism. Washington, DC, American Psychiatric Association Publishing, 2018

Kernberg OF: Psychotic personality structure. Psychodyn Psychiatry 47(4):353–372, 2019

Kernberg OF: Thoughts on transference analysis in transference-focused psychotherapy. Psychodyn Psychiatry 49(2):178–187, 2021

Loewald H: On the therapeutic action of psycho-analysis. Int J Psychoanal 41:16–33, 1960

Tuckett D: Does anything go? Int J Psychoanal 86:31–49, 2005

Tuckett D: Transference and transference interpretation revisited: why a parsimonious model of practice may be useful. Int J Psychoanal 100(5):852–876, 2019

Yeomans F, Clarkin JF, Kernberg OF: Transference Focused Psychotherapy for Borderline Personality Disorders: A Clinical Guide. Washington, DC, American Psychiatric Publishing, 2015

CHAPTER 4

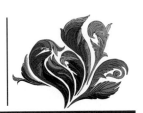

Therapeutic Implications of Transference Structures in Various Personality Pathologies

My main objective here is to illustrate the development of distinct organizations of transference presentations in various personality pathologies. These different transference developments are quite stable and consistent with neurotic, borderline, schizoid, narcissistic, and overtly psychotic patients and emerge in transference/countertransference developments in the context of psychoanalytic therapies. They are distinct, specific organizations of the internal world of object relations that determines the overall type or character of the personality. At the same time, I propose, they are a linkage between the concrete internal world of unconscious fantasy (the world of internalized instinctually—that is, affectively—invested object relations) and the structural aspects of character that distinguish personality types.

Reprinted from Kernberg OF: "Therapeutic Implications of Transference Structures in Various Personality Pathologies." *Journal of the American Psychoanalytic Association* 67(6):951–986, 2020. Used with permission.

Transference structures also have implications for the application of psychoanalytic technique. Certain aspects of psychoanalytic technique become prominent in particular therapeutic situations, for example, the importance of countertransference analysis, a required temporary relaxation of technical neutrality, or the need to focus sharply on specific aspects of the patient's external reality. I will clarify and illustrate these theoretical proposals, but first will examine some problems and possible misunderstandings raised by this extremely condensed overview.

First, with the term *transference structures* I refer to typical relationships between activated self- and object representations and their corresponding unconscious conflicts: it is not a matter of the content of specific unconscious fantasies evinced in individual sessions, which obviously are infinite in their highly individualized and unpredictable nature, but of the extent to which internal object relations reflect an integrated self, of whether self and internal objects are clearly differentiated from each other or are split to the degree that psychic experience is totally fragmented. Thus, I will be examining the structure of internalized object relations rather than the specific unconscious conflicts activated in each treatment session.

Second, whatever the predominant personality pathology of a patient, it is irrelevant for the utilization of a psychoanalytic understanding in each hour. Each session should be approached "without memory or desire." The degree and type of personality pathology is relevant for the overall possibility and indications for psychoanalysis and is related to overall prognosis (Kernberg 1999, 2018). In that new applications of modified psychoanalytic technique have expanded psychoanalysis with psychoanalytic psychotherapies for extremely disturbed patients, and that psychoanalysis and its derivative treatments are expanding the realm of psychoanalytic therapeutics, today personality theory/assessment and the expansion of psychoanalytic techniques are intimately related subject matters.

Third, in previous work I have attempted to define the body of what may be called "standard" or "classical" psychoanalytic technique as well as its modification for psychoanalytic psychotherapies (Kernberg 1999). More recently, in *Treatment of Severe Personality Disorders: Resolution of Aggression and Recovery of Eroticism* (Kernberg 2018), I outlined the corresponding differences in the application of psychoanalytic techniques.

I refer to "standard" or "classical" psychoanalytic technique as the approach to psychoanalytic treatment shared by the various schools or theoretical conceptions that today dominate our field: the ego psychological, Kleinian, British Independent, Relational, neo-Bionian, and (perhaps even) Lacanian approaches. This commonality is centered on the discovery and resolution of unconscious intrapsychic conflict by means of interpretation of defensive operations directed against unconscious impulses derived from libidinal and aggressive drives, conflicts activated dominantly in the transference. Transference analysis and the related exploration of correspondent countertransferences, carried out by the analyst from a predominantly neutral but not "indifferent" position, are the main instruments of this "standard" psychoanalytic technique. While modifications and expansions of this basic technique tend to be employed more freely in usual psychoanalytic practice, the Menninger study (Kernberg et al. 1972) found that the combination of specific modifications of these instruments may provide effective treatment for patients with severe psychopathology who do not respond well to psychoanalysis proper. This study showed that for patients with significant ego weakness, "expressive" psychotherapy with a combination of transference analysis and external support was more effective than psychoanalysis proper or supportive psychotherapy. In the Menninger project, Wallerstein (1986) found that some supportive techniques were quite frequently used in psychoanalysis proper, which led to their exploration in later work (Rockland 1989).

The Menninger study led to the development of a specific psychoanalytic psychotherapy, transference-focused psychotherapy (TFP; Kernberg 1975), the effectiveness of which could be empirically validated (Clarkin et al. 2007; Doering et al. 2010; Kernberg et al. 2008; Yeomans et al. 2015). Even a more differentiated, specific form of supportive psychotherapy has proved helpful, though less so than a truly psychoanalytic one. These findings signified an expansion of psychoanalytically based treatments that, independently, was researched in other centers (Rudolph 2013). In attempting to define the basic technical commonalities of psychoanalysis and psychoanalytic psychotherapies, and to clarify the differentiation of these approaches, I found interpretation, transference analysis, technical neutrality, and countertransference analysis to be the core psychoanalytic techniques that, combined in various degrees of modification, permit the definition of specific psychoanalytic psychotherapies (Kernberg 2018).

Interpretation involves the consistent analysis of defenses and of resistances as the clinical manifestations of these defensive operations. Transference analysis has emerged as a dominant therapeutic factor throughout the entire spectrum of psychoanalytic psychotherapies. Technical neutrality has been differently applied in alternative psychoanalytic approaches and is a major differentiating aspect of them. Countertransference analysis has raised the question of whether it should be communicated to the patient and, if so, to what extent. Countertransference "utilization" refers to the internal process of the analyst, not to its communication to the patient. Analytic understanding of the transference/countertransference dynamic includes the attention to the related, "intersubjective field."

Careful exploration of other leading technical psychoanalytic aspects (e.g., character analysis, dream analysis, enactment and acting out, working through, containment and reverie, repetition compulsion, negative therapeutic reaction, somatization, termination) reveals that they are applications of the four basic techniques of interpretation, transference analysis, technical neutrality, and countertransference (Kernberg 2018).

Fourth, it may rightly be questioned whether one can speak at this time of a "classical" or "standard" psychoanalytic technique, given the many psychoanalytic schools and orientations flourishing today. I have spelled out my own approach (Kernberg 2004b) and characterize it as a combined ego psychological and object relations approach that is very close to or integrated with a Kleinian perspective. In my efforts to arrive at a general definition of psychoanalytic technique, however, I have reached for broad technical definitions that incorporate relational perspectives as well. In the course of what follows, I comment on interventions that may raise questions from a Kleinian or relational perspective and clarify my reasons for making them. Regarding Kleinian perspectives, my work and that of my colleagues is quite close to Betty Joseph's approach to transference interpretation but includes additional observations regarding the object relation involved in projective identification and an expansion of the concept of total transference (Joseph 1985). Regarding the relational psychoanalytic approach, a major issue is the interpretation and management of countertransference developments, particularly with severely disturbed patients. I will illustrate what such dialogue with a relational approach would imply.

Fifth, to illustrate the activation, and transformation during the course of treatment, of characteristic transference structures in different psychopathologies, I will attempt to present the development of treatment over time. In illustrating with case material the various types of therapeutic structure developments, I will be limited in presenting the individual therapeutic hours of each case, thus limiting the process material that is always of highest interest to psychoanalysis. Despite these limitations, I hope to convey at least some process development that will illustrate my own analytic work and that of other colleagues.

Sixth, and finally, it is gratifying for a psychoanalyst that the work of the Cornell Personality Disorders Institute and of other dedicated psychoanalytic researchers has been effective in alerting the psychiatric community to the centrality of the nature of the self and its relations with significant others as the basis for classifying the severity of personality disorders, as reflected by Criterion A of the "Alternative DSM-5 Model for Personality Disorders" (American Psychiatric Association 2013). And in stressing the clinical relevance of the specific personality disorders that emerge in the psychoanalytic psychotherapies with them, psychoanalysis is pointing to the need to combine categorical criteria with dimensional (severity) considerations. I hope that these remarks will clarify the complexity that follows.

Classical psychoanalytic theory proposed that the symptoms of neurotic constellations and character pathology derive from unconscious infantile conflicts between drives and defensive operations. In the simplest terms, psychoanalytic treatment could be described as the systematic interpretation of defensive mechanisms to permit the gradual emergence into consciousness of the previously repressed drive derivatives in all their symptomatic expressions. This would permit a subsequent elaboration by the conscious ego, in the light of the adult capacity for integration and sublimation, of impulses not previously tolerated, as well as the related resolution of symptom formation.

Contemporary object relations theory has reformulated these basic psychoanalytic concepts in terms of the analysis of both drive derivatives and defensive operations as reflecting the internalization of relationships between self and others under the dominance of peak affect states representing these drive derivatives and defensive impulses (Fairbairn 1954; Greenberg and Mitchell 1983; Jacobson 1964; Kernberg 1985, 2004a, 2004b; Klein 1946, 1958; Winnicott 1965). In other words, rather than defining, for example, an obsessive character trait of excessive amiability as a compromise formation between an unconscious aggressive impulse and a defensive reaction formation directed against it, psychoanalytic object relations theory assumes that the aggressive impulse is constituted, in fact, by an aggressively framed internalized relationship between a dangerous, hostile object representation and an enraged self-representation. The corresponding defensive mechanism of surface friendliness reflects an internalized object relation involving a submissive self-representation relating to a powerful but protective and benign object representation. Both impulse and defense are represented by corresponding internalized object relations. Psychoanalytic technique, from an object relation theory viewpoint, now consists essentially in the systematic interpretation of both defensive and impulsive internalized object relations as they are reflected in the patient's pathological interactions with significant others, particularly in the transference.

The transference constitutes the optimal field in which these repressed or dissociated internalized object relations are activated, with the analyst and the patient assuming, in the patient's experience, the roles of the corresponding self- and object representations both defensive and impulsive. The predominant affect in their interaction reflects the underlying fantasized interaction between self and object that is being enacted in the transference. Within this framework, psychoanalytic technique can be defined as the systematic interpretation of the defensive internalized object relations represented by the defensive aspects of the transference, to be followed by the gradually predominant activation of the impulsive object relationship in the transference.

Freud observed that all that we know about drives are representations and affects; in the light of contemporary object relations theory, we might say that drives are represented by the dyadic relations between self- and object representations framed by a significant libidinal or aggressive "positive" or "negative" affect. These units are the building blocks of intrapsychic life. Eventually, they consolidate into ego, super-ego, and id as overall integrated structures, but at the same time their component discrete units of activated self- and object representations constitute transference dispositions that are the object of concrete inter-pretive interventions by the analyst.

The application of object relations theory to the study of psychic de-velopment has revealed the structural developments of two major stages of psychic life: first, an early stage of intrapsychic development in which internalized object relations are sharply dissociated or split according to their positive, rewarding or negative, aversive characteristics (Kernberg 1985; Kernberg and Caligor 2005). The temperamentally given, positive affect systems of eroticism, attachment, and play bonding, which may be viewed as jointly constituting the libidinal drive, are sharply split from the negative affect dispositions represented by the fight/flight and the separation-panic systems that jointly may be considered to represent the aggressive death drive (Panksepp and Biven 2012). The sharp splitting of internalized object relations, depending on the positive or negative af-fect systems that have been activated, determines a lack of integration of a total self and a lack of integration of total representations of significant others, so that idealized and devalued aspects of the self are dissociated, as well as idealized and persecutory aspects of significant others.

This early stage of development constitutes the condition described by the Kleinian school as the *paranoid-schizoid position*, and what has been defined more recently as the early developmental stage of identity dif-fusion (Kernberg 2012). Pathological fixation at this stage is the funda-mental structural characteristic of borderline personality organization (BPO). Under normal circumstances, a second stage of development gradually sets in over the first few years of life, characterized by inte-gration of the self, which now incorporates both positive and negative self-representations, and integration of the internalized representation of objects, with both the idealized and the persecutory aspects of signif-icant others being "toned down" into more realistic representations. This combination of an integrated self, surrounded by an integrated world of significant others, constitutes normal identity, characteristic of both normality and neurotic personality organization.

While contemporary object relations theory views all defense mech-anisms, as well as impulse-driven behavior, as corresponding to under-lying defensive and impulsive internalized object relations, a major difference at the borderline level, in contrast to a neurotic level of person-ality organization, is reflected in the predominance of primitive defen-sive operations centering around splitting, with consciously available but affectively split internalized object relations, idealized and persecu-tory, representing, respectively, defense and underlying impulse. The in-terpretation of the defensive operations at the borderline level deals with defensive and impulsive relations alternatively conscious and sharply split from each other activated in the transference.

In the case of neurotic personality organization, defense centers around repression and its related advanced defensive operations. This implies the interpretation of unconscious developments in the transference as unconscious elements of both defensive and of impulsive activation and justifies the classical view of the interpretation of unconscious impulsive contents on the basis of a previous elaboration of the defensive preconscious and unconscious defenses. In all cases, however, psychoanalytic technique implies, in essence, the interpretation of internalized object relations, particularly, but not exclusively, in transference activation, and the related use of clarification, confrontation, and interpretation proper of the corresponding object relationship between self- and object representations under the impact of a dominant affect state. Unconscious conflicts always emerge in the treatment situation as conflicts between a "defensive" self and object relations enacted with role distribution between analyst and patient, and "impulsive" self and object relations enacted in the transference. In all cases, analysis of the transference permits us to identify the corresponding unconscious conflicts, link the corresponding distorted interactions in the transference to parallel problems in the patient's external reality, and eventually trace them back into the patient's unconscious past.

Thus, the essential aspects of psychoanalytic technique across the entire spectrum of borderline and neurotic personality organization involve interpretation—with the differential features that interpretation takes in cases with normal identity or identity diffusion. As the term implies, transference analysis refers to the analysis of the dominant scenario of activation of past conflictual internalized object relationships as they appear in the interaction with the analyst. From a position of technical neutrality, the analyst describes the conflicts activated in the transference from a "third, excluded party" viewpoint. Such a position of technical neutrality, however, does not deny the importance of the activation of countertransference reactions and, on the contrary, uses the analysis of countertransference as part of the internal clarification of the transference by the analyst. Countertransference is used as an important, at times crucial, aspect of the information, including verbal and nonverbal communications by the patient, that permits transference interpretation. As mentioned, I have proposed elsewhere (Kernberg 2018) that these four technical interventions—interpretation, transference analysis, technical neutrality, and countertransference utilization—may be considered the basic techniques of psychoanalysis and psychoanalytic psychotherapy, and, in their systematic use throughout all psychoanalytic modalities of treatment, constitute the essence of psychoanalytic technique.

It should be added that to systematically employ psychoanalytic technique, including the four basic technical instruments and their derivative technical interventions, a certain therapeutic setting must be established that permits the development of the transference and the gradual deepening of the nature of therapeutic information and interventions. This setting of the therapeutic interaction is constituted by the clinician's maintaining him- or herself in an attitude of evenly suspended attention, and by the patient's being instructed to carry out free association. Again, this is not the place to analyze in detail the implications of the analyst's technical position and the importance of free association by the patient, but suffice it to say that establishment of the therapeutic frame will facilitate the activation of all the technical interventions I have mentioned.

In addition to the four basic analytic techniques, we may add the basic supportive techniques that, in contrast to analytic exploration, tend to reinforce the patient's defensive operations and compromise formations that may facilitate immediate improvement and adaptation to internal and external reality. In other words, if we add the techniques of supportive psychotherapy, which are often combined with analytically derived therapies, we will then have a list of all the psychoanalytically derived techniques and use it as a potential profile that allows the differential description and classification of the entire spectrum of psychotherapeutic approaches derived from, and including, standard psychoanalysis. These supportive techniques include abreaction, cognitive support, affective support, direct environmental intervention, and reeducational reduction of transference distortions as learning experiences to be transferred "outside" to the patient's external reality. This profile permits to us differentiate among the principal applications of psychoanalytic approaches, standard psychoanalysis, TFP, mentalization-based therapy, general psychodynamic psychotherapy, and supportive psychotherapy (Table 4–1).

Technical Implications of the Structural Aspects of the Transference

The original development of psychoanalytic technique occurred in the context of the predominant treatment of patients with neurotic personality organization. In other words, the various symptomatic conditions and character pathology focused upon by standard psychoanalysis and derived psychoanalytic psychotherapies were presented by a relatively healthier segment of the population, where standard psychoanalysis was the treatment of choice. In more recent times, the extension of psychoanalytic approaches to BPO, the severe personality disorders, and their complications (including alcoholism and addictions, perversions or "paraphilias," and severely regressed patients with borderline, narcissistic, schizoid, paranoid, and hypochondriacal pathology) has extended

Table 4–1. Dominant techniques in psychoanalytic psychotherapies

	Psychoanal	TFP	DPHP	TPOPSY	MBT	Ex-SupP	SPY
Interpretation	+++	+++	++	++	+	++	−
Transference analysis	+++	+++	++	+	+	+	−
Technical neutrality	+++	+−	+++	+	+	+	−
Countertransference utilization	++	+++	++	++	++	++	++
Abreaction	−	−	−	+	−	+	++
Cognitive support	−	−	−	+	+	+	+++
Affective support	−	−	−	+	+	+	+++
Environmental intervention	−	−	−	+	−	+	+++
Transference reduction and export	−	−	−	−	+	−	++

DPHP=dynamic psychotherapy for higher personality pathology; Ex-SupP=expressive-supportive psychotherapy; MBT=mentalization-based psychotherapy; Psychoanal=psychoanalysis; SPY=supportive psychotherapy; TFP=transference-focused psychotherapy; TPOPSY=German depth psychology–oriented psychotherapy.
Reprinted from Kernberg OF: "Therapeutic Implications of Transference Structures in Various Personality Pathologies." *Journal of the American Psychoanalytic Association* 67(6):951–986, 2020. Used with permission.

our knowledge to archaic psychic functions and structures. It has expanded our experience with regressive transference developments that require particular modifications of psychoanalytic treatment, modifications derived from the particular constellation of their respective transferences, and the technical implications evolving on that basis. In what follows, I will describe some structures of these regressive transference organizations and their technical implications, contrasting them with the typical transferences of neurotic personality organization.

NEUROTIC PERSONALITY ORGANIZATION: THE CLASSIC PSYCHOANALYTIC TREATMENT SITUATION

Classical psychoanalytic technique dealt primarily with patients presenting normal integration of identity, that is, an integrated concept of self, surrounded, we might say, by integrated concepts of significant others. This structure, within contemporary object relations theory, corresponds with the achievement of the depressive position, the integration of the persecutory and idealized segments of early experience into integrated concepts of self and others. It also involves full development of the tripartite structure of ego, superego, and id; a tolerance of ambivalence; and a capacity for deep and mature object relations (Kernberg and Caligor 2005). Most patients with hysterical, obsessive-compulsive, or depressive-masochistic personality structures fit this condition and, in the treatment, present typical development of regressive transferences involving the infantile self relating to various dominant infantile transference objects (Figure 4–1) (Caligor et al. 2007). Within these regressive transferences the patient usually incorporates his infantile self in a defensive or impulsive relationship with a significant infantile object projected onto the analyst. Analysis of this transference proceeds by gradually exploring and resolving the corresponding unconscious conflicts, preoedipal and oedipal, involved in their defensive and impulsive relationships. The patient's communication is mostly through verbal communication, although nonverbal communication, somatization, and acting out may at times prevail. Countertransference rarely acquires the role of a primary, overwhelming source of information regarding transference developments, though it is always present as important information.

To illustrate clinically: a woman in her mid-forties with an hysterical personality structure and significant masochistic features initially developed a regressive transference as part of which the analyst was experienced as a rigid, demanding, controlling figure representing the patient's mother. The patient experienced a sense of deep resentment for

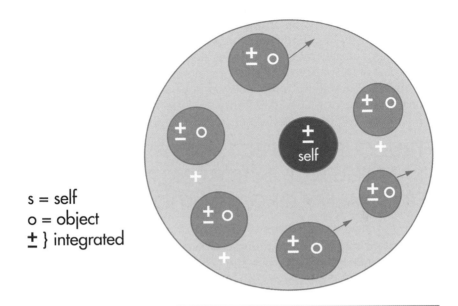

s = self
o = object
± } integrated

Figure 4–1. Neurotic transference.

Source.   Reprinted from Kernberg OF: "Therapeutic Implications of Transference Structures in Various Personality Pathologies." *Journal of the American Psychoanalytic Association* 67(6):951–986, 2020. Used with permission.

being oppressed and rebellious competitive impulses toward the analyst-mother. After a period of gradual working through, that dominant transference was replaced by the patient's activation of the relationship with a loving but weak and unreliable father who was unable to protect the patient and take her side in what she had experienced as unfair treatment by her mother. Still later, the transference evolved into a resentful and derogatory attitude toward the analyst, now perceived as hypocritical in his friendly "fatherly" demeanor while being emotionally unavailable. In a later stage of her analysis, and after working through enormous fears of experiencing forbidden sexual impulses toward him, the early image of a powerful and sexually provocative father emerged, with both erotic impulses in the transference and the fear of being rejected and depreciated, deeply connected with a fantasied sense of inferiority as a woman incapable of competing with powerful, dominant women ("mother"). This rather simplified and condensed history of the development of the dominant transference patterns of this analysis reveals, however, the continuity of the patient's self-concept throughout time, the projection of her temporarily corresponding object representations onto the analyst, and the relative stability of the self-concept in terms of the patient's maintaining a certain capacity for self-reflection throughout the entire treatment. This integrated self permitted her to explore, within the psychoanalytic setting, the particular unconscious conflictual relationships activated in the treatment situation.

The intensity of countertransference reaction was relatively moderate throughout the treatment. A consistently present "observing ego" on the part of the patient, and the correspondent capacity in the analyst to maintain a consistent "split" between specific countertransference responses and the ongoing availability of his self-reflecting function signaled the availability of a relatively stable therapeutic alliance.

STRUCTURAL ASPECTS OF THE TRANSFERENCE IN BORDERLINE PERSONALITY ORGANIZATION

In the psychoanalytic treatment of BPO, the typical structure of the transference implies a sharp division between the idealized and the persecutory segments of early psychic experience and the corresponding internalized object relations, with activation in the transference of split idealized and persecutory relationships (Kernberg 2004b). Here the lack of an integrated concept of self and the intensity of primitive affects facilitate the rapid activation of these split object relationships, reflected in the alternation of such intensely positive and negative transference reactions, not only the corresponding unconscious conflicts but, at the same time, rapid role reversals in their expression. Self- and object representations are interchanged in the transference. Alternately, at times the patient experiences himself to be a victim of the therapist's aggression, only then to make the therapist the victim of an aggressive transference. At other times, the therapist appears as an ideal, protective object, and the patient experiences himself in blissful dependency on such an object. This relationship, too, tends to alternate, with times in which the patient appears in the role of a giving mother and the therapist is placed in that of a happy, satisfied child, only to revert rapidly to the earlier persecutory relationship (Figure 4–2).

In this emotionally intense, rapidly shifting activation of contradictory affective states and corresponding object relations, what may initially present as an apparent chaos that may only gradually may be clarified, patients do not evince a basic, integrated self that would permit them to reflect on these activated states. These split object relations may only be integrated gradually, as the patient's understanding of his double identification with self and object and of their relationships grows, with the corresponding understanding that the projection of these split-off, chaotic internal relationships onto relationships with others in present reality is the source of the chaos, regression, and failure the patient has experienced.

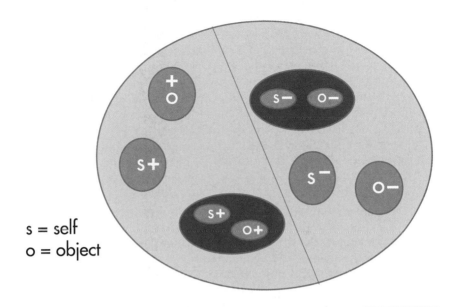

s = self
o = object

Figure 4–2. Borderline transference.

Source.   Reprinted from Kernberg OF: "Therapeutic Implications of Transference Structures in Various Personality Pathologies." *Journal of the American Psychoanalytic Association* 67(6):951–986, 2020. Used with permission.

TFP (Yeomans et al. 2015) has developed a specific technical approach that focuses on the dominant object relation in the transference at any point of the treatment, using the affectively dominant experience of the patient to diagnose the correspondent self- and object representations. The therapist pursues the activation of these relationships in the transference throughout time, diagnoses and interprets the sharp split between the idealized and the persecutory relation to the same infantile object, and thus attempts to integrate the self and the concepts of significant others, fostering the development of normal identity. Kleinian literature has stressed the fundamental function of projective identification in the attribution of internal object representations or internal self-experiences to significant others, particularly in the transference. But the Kleinian approach usually does not stress an activation of the *total object relationship*, with enactment of one aspect of this dyad by the patient, while the complementary object (or self) is projected onto the analyst (Spillius and O'Shaughnessy 2012).

The following case illustrates this transference structure in the psychoanalytic psychotherapy of a woman in her early twenties with borderline personality disorder and chronic, severe suicidal tendencies, sexual promiscuity, drug abuse, and failure in her studies. A central issue in her early childhood was the severe physical abuse she was chronically subjected by a maternal aunt, which her absent father passively tolerated. She initially displayed intense hostile reactions when her expectations and immediate wishes were not satisfied. Verbal attacks on the therapist escalated into attacks on objects in his office that required establishing rules limiting the patient's destructive behavior in the sessions. At other times, the patient bitterly complained about the indifference and coldness of the therapist, his sadistic pleasure, as she saw it, in frustrating her needs, complaining to third parties about the mistreatment by the analyst. Sometimes she presented rapid shifts between aggressive teasing, making fun of the therapist, provocatively sitting on his desk, and desperately crying when asked to leave at the end of the session; she would say she didn't have enough time to express something really important to her. At other times, through desperate pleas for phone contact and requests to increase the number of sessions, she showed intense wishes to depend on the therapist. She expressed fantasies that if the therapist were a kangaroo she would be his kangaroo baby, sitting in his pouch and watching, in a reassured mood, the world pass by. At one point, learning about a sudden catastrophe in the life of the therapist, the patient became extremely concerned, arriving to her session with a huge bunch of flowers, showing a role of maternal empathy and consolation to what she thought was the suffering therapist. It was only in the advanced stages of this treatment that the patient was able to tolerate the emotional awareness of both idealized and persecutory reactions to the therapist, experienced guilt over her aggressive behavior toward him, and wished to repair the damage that, in her fantasy, she might have caused him.

This may be the typical case where the intensity of acting out may induce a corresponding intensity of countertransference reactions, creates the threat of countertransference acting out, and poses the general question of how to deal with this development. This patient's intense rage and frustration when I did not satisfy her demands for time, attention, or special privileges coincided with her perception of me as a sadistic, withholding, torturing object: I became the aunt, and the patient was totally convinced that I behaved like that aunt. The patient was my helpless, suffering, enraged victim. And while I attempted to maintain the therapeutic boundaries, I could experience the pleasurable refusal to give in to her demands. To the contrary, when the patient attacked me viciously, insulting me on one occasion in a public space, on another destroying objects in my office, I felt the helpless victim of undeserved savagery: now she became the aunt, and I became the patient as the young, abused girl.

My technical approach consisted in clarifying, at the same time, who I represented in her massive projective identification, and who she was identifying with in her response to that projected object. The enacted transference/countertransference relationship was that between a sadistic aunt and an enraged, helpless, desperate child. At times, she experienced herself as a sadistic aunt in the transference, enacted this identification, and I became a helpless, enraged child in my countertransference. At other times, the relationship inverted to her experiencing herself as a helpless, mistreated child, while I became the vengeful, sadistic aunt. Through my interpreting this repeated reversal in our roles, the patient became able to understand her unconscious identification with both victim and perpetrator. The activation of this same object relation with role reversals between self and object in the transference made it possible, over time, to permit the patient to tolerate her unconscious identification with both self and object and recognize in herself what previously could only be projected. Thus, countertransference analysis and utilization in the context of the analysis of rapidly shifting transferences permits the patient eventually to understand also what is going on in the analyst during such intense interactions, without having to communicate to the patient the countertransference reaction as it occurs. This technical approach, I believe, is different from the relational approach of communicating intense countertransference developments to the patient as they evolve, and it may add to the Kleinian interpretation of projective identification in focusing sharply on the patient's experienced reaction to the analyst perceived under the effect of intense projective identification. "While you see me as sadistically commanding you around, you experience yourself as my helpless, impotent, enslaved victim." The central focus is on helping the patient understand the activation of the self and object relationships.

There are cases in which the severity of acting out will require limit setting to protect the structure of the treatment, thus threatening technical neutrality. Technical neutrality may temporarily be relaxed or abandoned altogether but must then be interpretively reinstated. These developments require the therapist to carry out very intense and ongoing internal work with powerful countertransference reactions typical in response to the activation of primitive transference developments in the treatment situation. While borderline patients may not tolerate a standard psychoanalytic setting, the flexibility of TFP permits systematic use of the four basic analytic techniques, so that these patients are provided a psychoanalytic treatment within a setting different from that of standard psychoanalysis.

STRUCTURAL ORGANIZATION OF THE TRANSFERENCE IN NARCISSISTIC PERSONALITY DISORDERS

Another type of typically structured transference developments is encountered with narcissistic personality disorder. Narcissistic personalities function at a broad level of pathology, with indication for standard psychoanalysis for those who evince a relatively normal capacity for work and/or a stable, if superficial, love relationship in the context of an ordinary social life (Kernberg 2004b, 2014). At the pathological extreme, severely regressed narcissistic personalities present with a total breakdown of their capacity to work or to maintain any intimate love relationship. They show a typical combination of absence of tenderness or emotional involvement in the context of intense sexual urges and promiscuity, with a concomitant breakdown in their social life. The most severely regressed narcissistic personalities are often diagnostically confused, at least initially, with regressed patients presenting a borderline personality disorder. Careful mental status examination usually reveals the presence of a pathological grandiose self, the essential clinical characteristic of this personality disorder.

The transference structure of narcissistic personality disorder presents a very typical development that persists stubbornly throughout months of psychoanalysis or psychoanalytic psychotherapy. It reflects the typical relation between the enactment of a pathological grandiose self and a projected condensation of the devalued, worthless aspects of the self and the devalued, worthless aspects of significant others (Figure 4–3). Here, the transference development appears as a relation between an omnipotent, omniscient grandiose self, and the devalued self-representation, usually projected onto the therapist, but with an ever threatening role reversal. The feared transference reversal then projects the grandiose self onto the therapist, while the patient enacts the devalued self-concept. The grandiose self does not relate to internalized valued object representations but exists in a strange isolation. Its only requirement, which is essential, is the admiration of significant others, needed to reconfirm its grandiosity and ensure its survival. Admiring objects, including the therapist in the transference, may be briefly idealized in an effort to incorporate that which is admirable in them and potentially envied in others, but are devalued and depreciated once they are not needed to implicitly confirm the pathological grandiose self. These developments dominate the transference for extended periods. Occasionally, the patient's objective failure in reality or in fantasy that he cannot deny brings about a sudden reversal of the relationship, so that the patient projects his grandiose self onto the therapist while identifying himself with the devalued self-representation usually projected onto others. By now it is well known how these grandiose, self-centered individuals suddenly become extremely insecure and dependent on reassurance from others in their social environment, only to rapidly revert to their original position of grandiosity.

In the transference, this pattern is enacted in a controlling and devaluing attitude toward the therapist, while attempts are made to maintain the therapist in a condition of sufficient appreciation to avoid consider-

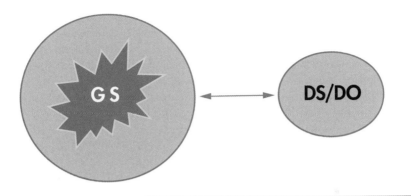

Figure 4–3. Narcissistic transference.

Source.   Reprinted from Kernberg OF: "Therapeutic Implications of Transference Structures in Various Personality Pathologies." *Journal of the American Psychoanalytic Association* 67(6):951–986, 2020. Used with permission.

ing the treatment totally useless. An authentic respect, interest, and appreciation for the therapist, to the contrary, would be dangerous, putting the patient immediately in a position of intolerable inferiority. At the origin of the structure of the grandiose self lies an internalization of what these patients experienced in early childhood as powerful and admired aspects of significant others, and their identification with aspects of themselves fostered in a parental environment in which admiration for a strikingly positive feature of the child replaced authentic love and concern on the part of the parents.

These component features that have activated the pathological grandiose self will gradually emerge, and in positive therapeutic developments this will allow that self to gradually decompose into its component idealized self- and object representations. This development will, in turn, activate the corresponding primitive object relations in the transference, idealized and persecutory split off from each other, and transform the narcissistic structure into a generally borderline one, a fundamental step toward improvement. When, as the pathological grandiose self is dismantled, component object representations are activated that reflect an identification with unethical aspects of parental images, these patients may evince antisocial features and dishonesty in the transference, which may complicate the development of normal superego functions in advanced stages of treatment. These are cases that present psychopathic transferences, which must be gradually transformed into predominantly paranoid transferences by analyzing the paranoid fears lying behind patients' dishonesty. Paranoid transferences may then be interpretively transformed into predominantly depressive transferences, in the context of identity integration.

But even when such complicating antisocial conditions are not present, the systematic analysis and decomposition of the pathological grandiose self usually takes months of "microanalysis" of the subtle ways in which the corresponding transference developments evolve. Subtle yet intense enactments of regressive part object relations occur as the pathological grandiose self is dismantled and carry a risk that the analyst will attribute the enactments of his countertransference reactions to "here-and-now" interactional processes, neglecting the profound early object relations being replayed in the transference.

To illustrate, I offer the case of a successful biological researcher, a man in his early fifties, effective, dominant, and controlling in complex business affairs but with no close friendships, a rather isolated social life, and a loveless marriage characterized by total sexual indifference. Chronic sexual promiscuity evincing little tenderness was his dominant source of sexual pleasure. He treated his wife like a slave who looked after his daily needs. In recent years she had gradually rebelled against this situation, expressed growing unhappiness with the empty nature of their marriage, and finally had told her husband she was considering divorce. At that point, an anxious collapse of the patient's grandiosity brought him to treatment, initially to deal with the marital conflict, which rapidly turned out to reflect deep problems in his sexual life and social interactions. He was diagnosed with narcissistic personality disorder, with psychoanalysis the treatment of choice.

He quickly developed a transference with the characteristics described above. He considered the analyst a mediocre, small-thinking "technician" who was trying to apply the book, knowledge that the patient, on the basis of his readings, felt he had himself possessed all along. An ongoing complaint was that he had been "conned into" a useless treatment. It took many months of treatment to open up an awareness of his defenses against intense envy of his wife's emotional richness and the gratification he felt the analyst must take in his work. The patient, by contrast, felt himself involved in a constant professional and financial competition in his work, which have him no rest or relaxation. Gradually, a very frustrating early childhood emerged, both parents being experienced by him as insensitive and unavailable; the gradual development of a sense of successful competition and triumphant superiority over schoolmates was the only source of gratification in his childhood. Eventually, components of his grandiose self could be isolated and explored in the transference.

The following example illustrates this development. The patient lived in the same professional environment as his analyst, a mid-size Midwestern city. He would attentively listen to any gossip that he could catch regarding his analyst, eventually constructing a story about supposedly inappropriate and ridiculous behavior by his analyst that the patient then spread among acquaintances. This story made the rounds and finally came back to him: somebody told him the same story he had spread about me, the analyst. The patient, frightened by this, decided to "confess" to me that he was the source of this gossip. Despite intense negative countertransference, the analyst was able to maintain the analytic relationship and gradually, over a period of several weeks, analyze what had motivated this intensely invested behavior by the patient.

It turned out that it replicated the behavior of his mother, who, coming from a socially disadvantaged environment, chronically felt insecure in the socially privileged environment of her husband, the patient's father. The patient had a clear sense of his mother as frequently gossiping about her social acquaintances in order to diminish the importance of people she envied and felt insecure with. As an aspect of his pathological grandiose self, he had incorporated this image and source of power of his mother, now expressed in the transference relation with the analyst. By the same token, here the relationship between the patient's pathological grandiose self and the projected devalued self became transformed into the specific relation between the mother-identified patient and the projection of his neglected and rejected self-representation in the transference. In other words, this specific transference relationship heralded the dismantling of his pathological grandiose self. The patient now experienced authentic feelings of shame and guilt over his behavior, and it was a first recognition of the origin of aggression within himself, in contrast to its usual projection onto others.

I was quite shocked when I first became aware of the patient's spreading gossip about me. My first reaction was the wish to terminate his treatment. I felt disappointed and betrayed, consulted with a senior colleague, and was able to maintain the treatment, but only with an inhibition in my interpretive interventions. I clearly became aware that the patient was identifying himself with his gossipy, envious, and depreciative mother, but it took me some time to realize that I was not simply reacting as the betrayed and abandoned son. I also developed a devaluating, vengefully superior reaction in my countertransference. Exploring with the patient his experience of me as superior and devaluating, and his shameful sense of having to depend on such an object, clarified for me why having put me down outside the sessions was a relieving reversal of the situation. Again, I was able to help him understand his identification with both self and object in this conflictual, highly traumatic experience, as well as the related defensive function of his grandiosity.

STRUCTURAL ORGANIZATION OF THE TRANSFERENCE IN SCHIZOID PERSONALITY DISORDERS

The concept of schizoid transferences lends itself to confusion because of two different uses of this concept. The classical psychiatric definition of the schizoid personality disorder clearly describes the characteristic symptoms that lend themselves to diagnostic assessment and that indeed are fundamental for assessing typical schizoid transference dispositions that have been relatively underappreciated in the psychiatric literature. At the same time, the Kleinian concept of the paranoid-schizoid position (Klein 1946), based in part on the description of the psychodynamics of the schizoid position elaborated by Fairbairn (1954), has dominated the psychoanalytic literature and proven itself essential in the analysis of the defensive organization of the entire field of BPO, that is, the defensive dissociation or split between idealized and persecutory internalized object relations. Paranoid-schizoid dynamics are found in the entire field of patients with severe personality disorders but are to be differentiated from the very specific transferences that characterize the schizoid personality disorder, which require a specific technical approach originally suggested by Fairbairn (1954), Guntrip (1969), and Rey (1979). These specific transference dispositions described by Fairbairn correspond more closely to the classical psychiatric concept of the schizoid and schizotypal personality disorders.

Typical descriptive characteristics of the schizoid personality disorder include social withdrawal, social isolation, a lack of intimate relationships, hypersensitivity to criticism, feeling very easily hurt by others, and a particular, heightened sensitivity to the feelings and behavior of others, in contrast to these patients' social isolation (Akhtar 1992). At the same time, these patients seem to withdraw into a private, secretive self-affirmation and an internal world of fantasy that they control. This self-affirmation lacks the sense of superiority and depreciation of significant others that is characteristic of the pathological grandiose self of narcissistic personalities. The schizoid patients as described by Fairbairn present, as a dominant dynamic, a desperate desire for close, dependent relationships but, at the same time, an extraordinary fear of overwhelming control by the other, of being swallowed by any close relationship. In contrast to their lack of capacity for empathic and tender relationships with others, they frequently present a dissociated "explosion," the activation of sexualized and aggressive relationships in a dissociated mode.

They miss the modulated activation of affect dispositions and present a highly specific fragmentation or dispersal of affects. Positive and negative affects seem equally unavailable, except in sudden dissociated outbursts, in contrast to a chronic, apparent unavailability of explicit affective experiences. These patients evince, as a predominant structure, a fragmented sense of self—that is, a disturbing, confusing unawareness of their present affective self experience, which contrasts with the alternating activation of idealized and persecutory affective experiences of ordinary borderline patients. Schizoid patients' experiences of significant others are equally fragmented. They find it difficult to divide the

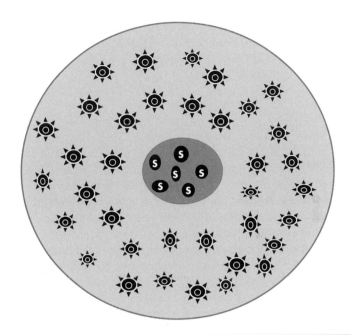

Figure 4–4. Schizoid transference.

Source. Reprinted from Kernberg OF: "Therapeutic Implications of Transference Structures in Various Personality Pathologies." *Journal of the American Psychoanalytic Association* 67(6):951–986, 2020. Used with permission.

world into idealized and persecutory objects: because of a great sensitivity regarding individual behaviors and interactions that defy a clear differentiation between "positive" and "negative" objects, they experience others in confusing ways. In other words, they experience fragmentation of affects rather than splitting mechanisms. From the viewpoint of Fairbairn's analysis, which includes both the descriptive, classical symptoms of the schizoid personality and their dominant dynamics, the assumption of a purely descriptive psychiatric approach that considers these patients as having no desire for intimate relationships clearly ignores their deeper psychological reality. Figure 4–4 presents the schizoid structural organization that manifests in the transference as an activation of these fragmented relationships, including the fragmentary self and the fragmentary experiences with others.

Practically, these patients appear to be very distant, with no specific affect activation in the sessions, thus confusing the therapist as to the dominant object relationship being enacted in the transference at any particular point. The therapist may feel confused about his affective reaction to the patient, which seems to center in the feeling of nonunderstanding or confusion about the situation, matched by the patient's indications of being similarly confused, having no clear sense of what it is all about and no clear sense of his own affective experiences. It is as if, in spite of, or due to, verbal communications with a trivial, impersonal, meaningless, or distracting quality, the affective relationship in the session remains strangely distant. The therapist's effort to clarify what is in the patient's mind may lead the patient to a sense of confusion, a feeling of being invaded, or, if the therapist tentatively suggests that a dominant present relationship seems to be activated, the patient may evince a frightened sense of being invaded, controlled, or brainwashed. The therapist may in turn easily feel that he has engaged in a theory-driven statement rather than doing justice to the dominant affective relationship. The solution to this situation of therapeutic uncertainty for the therapist lies in recognizing the relative failure of verbal communication regarding transference clarification and accepting the central function, under these conditions, of the activation of countertransference reactions.

Countertransference may provide answers if the therapist can let himself be influenced by the total situation in which he is now engaged with the patient. It is an intersubjective situation that cannot be traced back to any particular experience of patient or therapist but clearly reflects the nature of the atmosphere created by their actual interaction. This requires an openness by the therapist to the activation of whatever dominant affect state develops in him, an openness to the fantasies that may accompany such an affect state or that may seem the activators of a certain affect state, and the use of that dominant affect and the related fantasy material to reexamine the interaction with the patient in light of the patient's dominant pathology and his external reality at this point. That gradual, difficult, but feasible analysis may lead to an understanding of what affective relation is presently dominant while being dispersed and fragmented to an extent that initially made it impossible to gather.

Technically, here the same use of the four basic techniques applies, but with particular caution regarding interpretation and, even more so, transference interpretation. The therapist may venture interpretations that may be easily rejected by the schizoid patient, and the therapist must be prepared to accept such a rejection, with further exploration about what the patient thinks might be more applicable at the moment than what the therapist is saying. A willingness to retrace one's own observation, to share with the patient that one understands the patient's difficulty in clarifying what is going on in his mind, as a difficulty parallel to that of the therapist to clarify what is going on in the interaction, may be a helpful, reassuring assertion of uncertainty. It should not be difficult to differentiate this development from a narcissistic patient's contemptuous rejection of interpretations by the analyst. The therapist must therefore be cautious in interpreting the thinking of the schizoid patient and must stress his search for clarity in the patient's thinking, as well as in the therapist's own.

In this context, the patient's rejecting behavior and mistrust needs to be tolerated, as well as the indications of his hypersensitive reaction to a perceived rejection by the therapist. The patient may give indications of wanting to be close, being afraid of it, withdrawing in a suspicious attitude, and even a preventive explicit rejection of the therapist as a protection against excessively desired and feared closeness. The nature of the affectively dominant object relationship defended against by the prevalent schizoid fragmentation mechanism may vary widely: patients may reveal erotic fantasies behind the apparent emptiness of the session, intense fusional longings, or aggressive, dependent, paranoid affective dispositions, with variable condensations between oedipal and preoedipal relationships. The following case illustrates a prevalent schizoid transference.

The patient presented a typical schizoid personality disorder. A woman in her early twenties, she chronically cut herself with razor blades to observe the bleeding. She had evinced serious social isolation from early childhood on and a total social breakdown in college, where she could not relate to other students and where her withdrawal into an intense world of fantasies prevented her from concentrating on her studies. Clinically, the extent of her social withdrawal, her cutting off relationship with family and friends, the failure at school, her rapid withdrawal from several early dating experiences that seemed to cause traumatic reactions in her, and her almost disorganized way of talking raised the question whether she suffered from a schizophrenic illness. After extended psychiatric evaluations it became clear that she presented a schizoid personality disorder, and the treatment recommended was TFP.

In the first few weeks of treatment, after the usual history was taken, our interaction evolved into a superficial, almost mechanical repetitive communication of trivial aspects of her daily living. After the first 2 or 3 months of treatment, I started to find it almost impossible to concentrate on anything in the sessions with her or to use whatever cues seemed available to direct our interaction into some meaningful communication. My efforts to inquire into what she was feeling, what her fantasies were, led to more of the same trivial communications, and I could sense her irritation with me when she felt I was forcefully attempting to find new meanings in what she was saying. At the same time, she would come punctually to all sessions and seemed not to object to the empty content of what evolved in them. She referred vaguely to her tendency to cut herself discreetly and to watch drops of blood emerging. There was an occasional seductive quality about some of her expressive demeanor, so tentative and transitory that it was gone by the time I felt there was some significance in it.

I had occasional fantasies that she focused on the discreet cutting of her skin to observe blood drops as a way to exhibit herself to me or perhaps enact a fantasy of me attacking her sexually, or that I was a father figure who failed in protecting her, but all efforts to explore her world of fantasy led nowhere. It was as if whatever I said confused and disorganized her thinking, and my own thinking seemed to get confused at such moments. I pointed out to her that she experienced my efforts to understand her as invasive and that it was as if any attempt at clarification was dangerous.

In one session, I had great difficulty maintaining my attention on what she was saying. I was following my own thoughts and suddenly remembered a film I had seen 6 months earlier, *Investigation of a Citizen Beyond Suspicion*, an Italian film about a district attorney in charge of finding a sexual murderer. The district attorney, who was himself the murderer, would kill women in the process of having sex with them. One image from that film came to my mind. A woman reaching orgasm was sitting on top of that district attorney when he suddenly pulled out a knife and cut her throat, blood running over her breasts. This scene came into my mind, with a combination of excitement and disgust, followed by a kind of frightened surprise on my part that I should develop such a fantasy, and in the middle of such a session. I attempted to dismiss the memory of that experience over the next few days. But then I realized that her repetitive comments about her body, and bleeding openings, and the strangely seductive moments in the sessions with this extremely inhibited patient, and my sense of "shock" over my sadistic sexual fantasy, reflected an oscillating countertransference identification with both a self- and an object representation involved in a sadomasochistic interaction. And I understood that my frequent sense of confusion also represented the effect of the patient's defensive fragmentation of all emotional experiences. I said that there were threatening sexual thoughts "in the air" that could not be talked about.

Several weeks later, when the patient mentioned there were thoughts she had difficulty talking about, she referred to a powerful fantasy about me that she had had repeatedly. She wished I would shoot her, and in killing her become a murderer. I then would remain, for the rest of my life, feeling regretful. I would never be able to forget her, and she would remain with me the rest of my life. She would not mind dying, knowing she would be my permanent companion the rest of my life! This sexual fantasy, with regressive oedipal and severely aggressive preoedipal sadomasochistic and self-destructive implications, became a central focus of our exploration in the following months. What I want to stress here is the close relationship between what was developing in the transference and the nature of my countertransference fantasy in the middle of the apparently fragmented, dispersed activation of a specific object relationship. This example may seem unusual, but in fact it is a quite frequent type of experience in countertransference developments when the therapist tolerates the fragmented relationship of a schizoid transference. The opening up of a specific relationship gradually transforms the schizoid transference into the more usual transferences of BPO and makes the treatment much easier to carry out within the general technical approach for patients with identity diffusion. The specific defensive problem presented by this fragmentation or dispersal of affect raises an open question. Is this a purely psychological development of the intrapsychic world of these patients, or does it reflect a more basic neurobiological disposition to dispersal of particular, excessively intense negative affects?

STRUCTURAL ASPECTS OF SYMBIOTIC TRANSFERENCE DEVELOPMENTS

The term *symbiotic* has been used in ambiguous ways in the literature. In one use it refers to relationships in which an intense enmeshment between self and other would not tolerate another relationship to coexist with this particular enmeshed one. The boundary between self and other is maintained, but the relationship has an exclusive quality, no other relationship with a "third party" is tolerated, and exchange between self and other by means of projective identification facilitates alternative identification with self and other. The term's other use refers to actual merger between the concept of self and other, a relationship in which there evolves a lack of differentiation between self and other, so that self experience and experience of the other are confused, with the implicit loss of ordinary ego boundaries. In the second use of the term, an authentic psychotic process is present, and the loss of reality testing underlies the development of abnormal perceptions, hallucinations, and delusions. In contrast, in symbiotic relationships in which the differentiation between self and object always is maintained—although they are enmeshed, there may be very rapid interchange of roles between self and other. I am reserving the term *symbiotic transference* for an intense, entangled involvement between self and other, but with clear maintenance of boundaries between self and other, even when rapid exchange of the role relationship develops. I reserve the term *psychotic transference* for cases with loss of differentiation between self and other, a merger of self and other that implies the loss of ego boundaries and reality testing. Figure 4–5 outlines a symbiotic transference, in contrast to Figure 4–6, which depicts a psychotic transference.

In the ordinary activation of transferences typical of BPO, patients may tolerate intense differences of views with the therapist and express their conflicts in sharply differentiated roles within a specific affect-centered relationship between self- and object representations. In symbiotic relations, patients tolerate no difference between their view of re-

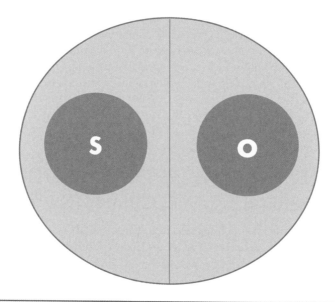

Figure 4–5. Symbiotic transference.

Source. Reprinted from Kernberg OF: "Therapeutic Implications of Transference Structures in Various Personality Pathologies." *Journal of the American Psychoanalytic Association* 67(6):951–986, 2020. Used with permission.

ality and that of the therapist. The therapist must agree totally with the patient. Any disagreement indicates either a violent invasion of the patient's mind by a therapist who disagrees with him or total abandonment by a therapist who ignores him and, by the same token, violently abandons him. Britton (2004) has described this situation as an intolerance of triangulation. We also see this development in some severely regressed borderline patients. The patient has no tolerance of the therapist's involvement with anyone else, with any other person or entity, or other ways of thinking, from which the patient would be excluded. This may reflect an archaic defense against an early oedipal situation, in which mother has to be totally identified with the baby, and the existence of mother's relationship with father has to be completely denied; or it may express intense envious resentment of the life, knowledge, and general existence of the therapist outside the realm of the patient's mind. In any case, only a primitive coincidence of thinking, or total and exclusive availability of the therapist to the patient in his mind, is tolerable. This is an ideal situation, against which any "betrayal" by the therapist's otherness triggers intolerable rage and resentment in the patient, who fears destructive invasion or total abandonment by this betrayal.

The clinical conditions under which such a development occurs are difficult to foresee, though usually this complication presents in patients

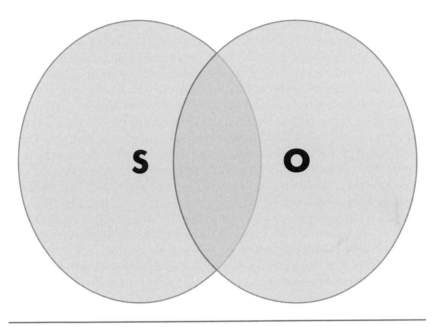

Figure 4–6. Psychotic transference.

Source.   Reprinted from Kernberg OF: "Therapeutic Implications of Transference Structures in Various Personality Pathologies." *Journal of the American Psychoanalytic Association* 67(6):951–986, 2020. Used with permission.

with an extreme incapacity to adjust to ordinary social interactions, who evince an intense aggression rationalized by projective identification and omnipotent control that severely distorts their intimate relationships. Once such a symbiotic transference becomes dominant, it can be recognized by its threatening character, the extended duration of a patient's incapacity to tolerate any contrary ideas in the therapist, desperate efforts by the patient to maintain control of reality under such conditions, and his apparent total incapacity to recognize ordinary logic. At this point the treatment must focus almost exclusively on this very development, the patient's incapacity to tolerate any difference of views and the reasons why such difference would develop panic in the patient.

The following example illustrates a symbiotic transference in a patient with the diagnosis of severe narcissistic personality disorder with overt borderline functioning, that is, almost total breakdown in the capacity for work, for intimate relations, and for an ordinary social life. She was a woman in her early forties, treated in a psychoanalytic psychotherapy by a skilled psychoanalyst. At one point one of her brothers died, which she experienced as a terrible blow. At the cemetery, while her brother was being buried, the patient broke out in intense crying and dramatic manifestations of intolerable psychic pain, approaching the

grave and looking as if she would throw herself in after the coffin. Naturally, she created quite a commotion. People were holding her back as she
became enraged and angrily accused her family of being insensitive to
her grief. She had to be escorted from the cemetery by family members.

In the psychotherapeutic session following this event, the patient was
still enraged, complaining about the insensitivity and brutality of her
family at the cemetery. The therapist first expressed his interest and understanding of the patient's emotional reaction. He clarified her sense of
rage over her family's lack of understanding and real feelings. Then,
when he asked how she understood the reactions to her at the cemetery,
she declared their behavior to have been completely inappropriate and
incomprehensible. The therapist tactfully tried to confront her with the
fact that it seemed, from everything he was aware of, that her behavior
had been rather inappropriate, disturbing the ceremony that was taking
place. To this she reacted with even more rage, accusing the therapist of
being in cahoots with her family, being totally insensitive, and having no
understanding of her. In short, he was a total disappointment. She wondered whether she could stay in treatment with him under these conditions. The therapist, realizing she was unable to reflect on this experience,
limited his intervention to expressing his understanding of her suffering,
with no further effort to clarify the situation at the cemetery. It took a
number of weeks, and many sessions, for the patient to consider the possibility that the therapist might have a different view of the situation at the
cemetery, even if she disagreed with him. It took even longer for her to
recognize or even consider that the therapist's might actually be valid.
Just her acceptance of the fact that the therapist might think differently,
without that signifying a total attack or rejection of the patient, became a
major issue to be explored in the treatment. In more general terms, this
case illustrates not only intolerance of triangulation—the therapist holding to another view—but also the patient's profound underlying incapacity to consider that she might be taken seriously, respected in her own
views, and appreciated by an early maternal object.

THE STRUCTURE IN
PSYCHOTIC TRANSFERENCES

Psychotic transference dispositions are characterized by a lack of differentiation between self- and object representations or a lack of differentiation between self and other that is reflected in the loss of reality testing.
This situation has been explored in the psychoanalytic literature and described in the experience of intensive psychoanalytic psychotherapy
with psychotic patients in the United States and the United Kingdom before the development of psychopharmacological medication, particularly in institutions dedicated to intense psychotherapeutic approaches
to psychosis. Harold Searles (1965) described intensive psychotherapy

with schizophrenic patients as undergoing typical stages: first, a stage of lack of contact or absence of a specific transference relationship; second, a stage of intense symbiotic development, evincing the lack of differentiation between self and other as the typical dynamic of intense psychotic transferences; third, a phase of differentiation, in which the patient gradually learns to differentiate himself from the therapist, with recovery of reality testing regarding his behavior and his contribution to the transference relationship. A fourth phase of integration follows in which the patient becomes able to integrate the mutually dissociated aspects of his earlier transference experiences and experiences a parallel integration of his sense of self and of the nature of the relationship with his therapist. This integration may then be generalized to other relationships of the patient. Herbert Rosenfeld (1954) applied a Kleinian perspective to the analysis of the confusional states and primitive (psychotic) mechanisms dominating clinical encounters with schizophrenic patients.

Due to pharmacological advances, intensive psychotherapy of psychosis has receded as an important treatment modality, but it may still be indicated for a subgroup of patients defined by Michael Stone (1983, 1986). These are schizophrenic patients who do not respond to psychopharmacological treatment with restoration of reality testing, have a high intellectual level, maintain a certain integration of the personality and significant differentiation of affect states, do not present antisocial features, and provide the possibility of intensive long-term treatment under the provision of a sufficiently structured environment to absorb unavoidable periods of acting out.

I once had the opportunity of treating an 18-year-old girl who suffered from paranoid schizophrenia, at a time when intensive psychotherapeutic treatment seemed an important aspect of the treatment of such conditions, when psychopharmacological treatment was still in its early experimental stages and had not yet evolved as the treatment of choice. I saw the patient under supervision in a highly regarded hospital specializing in this kind of treatment. In the first few months of the treatment I had to see her in a padded cell under constant nursing observation. This patient would tear up all her clothing and could only with great difficulty be made to wear anything on her body. She was sitting naked in the cell, masturbating much of the time, and smelling the fingers she had used in masturbating. When I entered the cell to see her, she ignored me completely and continued masturbating.

I need to stress that, in spite of her physical attractiveness and this open sexual behavior, there was a total lack of erotic quality in her demeanor and in the atmosphere of that room. It is difficult to describe, but there was a totally impersonal quality about the contact she established with me, as if I were some strange object rather than a human being. I was myself totally surprised by the lack of any erotic quality of her behavior or of the atmosphere she created in that cell. Her delusions were that the devil was forcing her to have sex and invading the world to force everybody to have sex with him. She was attempting to assure herself that the devil had not destroyed her genitals, while believing that her parents were being held prisoners by the devil, who had divided humanity into those who were in prison and those who would be sexually abused. It was a quite chaotic system of delusions, mixed with other fantasies and delusions involving nurses and teachers. I was trying to find the sense of all this delusional material, trying to formulate it to myself as clearly as I could, conveying an attitude of interest and effort to understand what was going on in her mind, and attempting to help her clarify whatever was confusing her. It was painful and laborious work, in the course of which I found her becoming more and more attentive to me but giving no indication that what I was saying influenced her in any way.

Only very gradually did I realize that she was evaluating whether I was in any way a secret representative or emissary of the devil and hiding that from her. Eventually we could talk about her suspecting me of not being honest and straightforward and that this seemed frightening to her. Then one day I entered her cell, and there was a clearly erotic atmosphere in the air. I couldn't decide what brought this about, but the patient clearly showed a seductive attitude toward me and looked at me sexually provocatively while still masturbating. She told me with a sardonic smile, "I am the devil and you are the devil," treating both of us as if we were the devil enjoying seducing her sexually. It was an intense and disturbing experience because she now really appeared sexually attractive to me, while at the same time I was afraid she would assault me. I was reassured by the fact that the windows of that room were constantly monitored by the nursing service.

My effort in the following sessions was to point out to the patient that the danger of being sexually assaulted by the devil had now taken the form of misdiagnosing "us" as the devil, rather than her simply being the victim and I an emissary from the devil. In other words, my effort went into attempting to differentiate two people out of what at that moment was a clear condensation of her experience of herself and of me: we both were the devil and the frightened girl. I believe this vignette illustrates the shift from an early phase of a psychotic transference ("symbiotic" in Searles' [1965] terminology) and my early efforts to help the patient move into the phase of differentiation between self- and object representation.

THE DEAD MOTHER SYNDROME: DISMANTLING TRANSFERENCES

A final type of specific transference disposition may be characterized as the dismantling of all internalized object relations and the correspondent implication of a radical emotional unavailability in the treatment: namely, the "dead mother syndrome" described by André Green (1993; Kohon 1999). Here the tragedy is the patient's lack of capacity for any investment in a significant relationship because of the unconscious protective dismantling of all internalized relationships. These patients usually present a very early traumatic background of an absent mother, often due to severe chronic depression in the mother during infancy or early childhood. In these cases the unconscious wish to become reunited with their mother in death is reflected in a sense that only the absence of all actual relationships will facilitate such a condition. These patients develop a dangerous lack of emotional investments despite otherwise normal intelligence, capacity to differentiate self from non-self, capacity for superficial yet adequate social and work relations, and surprisingly normal superego functions, so that the lack of emotional involvement becomes evident only in intimate contexts. Their extraordinary capacity to maintain an apparently friendly but insurmountable distance in the therapeutic relationship poses a major challenge over many months, even years, of treatment. These are, fortunately, very rare cases, with reserved prognosis, and are mentioned here only to contrast them with transference patterns determined by internalized object relations, patterns that require specific employment of the four basic psychoanalytic techniques. I will not explore these cases further here. The specific technical requirements and challenges of the "dead mother" syndrome have been explored elsewhere.

Concluding Comment

Classical psychoanalytic technique evolved in the context of Freud's work, primarily with neurotic patients, showing a predominance of an integrated tripartite intrapsychic structure, corresponding to normal identity. In light of the expansion of the spectrum of severity of patients' pathology being treated with psychoanalytic psychotherapy, as well as psychoanalysis, and experience with modifications of classical technical psychoanalytic instruments, we now have available a broad spectrum of psychoanalytically based techniques that, jointly, should permit their selective application across a broad spectrum of pathology. Standard psychoanalysis may now be described as a specialized, classical form of that body of techniques, offering a unique potential for further exploration of unconscious conflicts, defensive operations, and structural organization in both normal and pathological functioning. This classical technique is of central interest for psychoanalytic education and for teaching this standard technique for the treatment of neurotic patients. To some extent, these applications have already been subjected to empirical research that confirms the effectiveness of psychoanalytic approaches to severe personality disorders. At the same time, we may now consider the integrated body of psychoanalytic techniques as a broad spectrum of related technical interventions based on psychoanalytic theory that can be combined and modified according to the specific type of transference structures that reflect various degrees and types of personality organization and thus make psychoanalytic technique a body of instruments that have a broad spectrum of application in psychoanalytic psychotherapies.

References

Akhtar S: Broken Structures. Northvale, NJ, Jason Aronson, 1992

American Psychiatric Association: Diagnostic and Statistical Manual of Mental Disorders, 5th Edition. Arlington, VA, American Psychiatric Association, 2013

Britton R: Subjectivity, objectivity, and triangular space. Psychoanal Q 73:47–61, 2004

Caligor E, Kernberg OF, Clarkin JF: Handbook of Dynamic Psychotherapy for Higher Level Personality Pathology. Washington, DC, American Psychiatric Publishing, 2007

Clarkin JF, Levy KN, Lenzenweger MF, Kernberg OF: Evaluating three treatments for borderline personality disorder: a multiwave study. Am J Psychiatry 164: 992–998, 2007

Doering S, Horz S, Rentrop M, et al: Transference-focused psychotherapy v. treatment by community psychotherapists for borderline personality disorder: randomized controlled trial. Br J Psychiatry 196:389–396, 2010

Fairbairn W: An Object-Relations Theory of the Personality. New York, Basic Books, 1954

Green A: Le Travail du Négative. Paris, Editions de Minuit, 1993

Greenberg J, Mitchell S: Object Relations in Psychoanalytic Theory. Cambridge, MA, Harvard University Press, 1983

Guntrip H: Schizoid Phenomena, Object-Relations and the Self. New York, International Universities Press, 1969

Jacobson E: The Self and the Object World. New York, International Universities Press, 1964

Joseph B: Transference: the total situation. Int J Psychoanal 66:447–454, 1985

Kernberg OF: Borderline Conditions and Pathological Narcissism. New York, Jason Aronson, 1975

Kernberg OF: Internal World and External Reality: Object Relations Theory Applied. Northvale, NJ, Jason Aronson, 1985

Kernberg OF: Psychoanalysis, psychoanalytic psychotherapy and supportive psychotherapy: contemporary controversies. Int J Psychoanal 80:1075–1091, 1999

Kernberg OF: Aggressivity, Narcissism, and Self-Destructiveness in the Psychotherapeutic Relationship. New Haven, CT, Yale University Press, 2004a

Kernberg OF: Contemporary Controversies in Psychoanalytic Theory, Techniques, and Their Applications. New Haven, CT, Yale University Press, 2004b

Kernberg OF: Identity: recent findings and clinical implications, in The Inseparable Nature of Love and Aggression: Clinical and Theoretical Perspectives. Washington, DC, American Psychiatric Publishing, 2012, pp 3–30

Kernberg OF: An overview of the treatment of severe narcissistic pathology. Int J Psychoanal 95:865–888, 2014

Kernberg OF: The basic components of psychoanalytic technique and derivative psychoanalytic psychotherapies, in Treatment of Severe Personality Disorders: Resolution of Aggression and Recovery of Eroticism. Washington, DC, American Psychiatric Association Publishing, 2018, pp 49–72

Kernberg OF, Caligor E: A psychoanalytic theory of personality disorders, in Major Theories of Personality Disorder, 2nd Edition. Edited by Lenzenweger M, Clarkin JF. New York, Guilford, 2005, pp 114–156

Kernberg OF, Burstein ED, Coyne A, et al: Psychotherapy and Psychoanalysis: Final Report of the Menninger Foundation's Psychotherapy Research Project, Vol 36, No 1 and 2. Topeka, Kansas, Menninger Foundation, 1972

Kernberg OF, Yeomans F, Clarkin JF, Levy KN: Transference focused psychotherapy: overview and update. Int J Psychoanal 89(3):601–620, 2008

Klein M: Notes on some schizoid mechanisms. Int J Psychoanal 27:94–110, 1946

Klein M: On the development of mental functioning. Int J Psychoanal 39:84–90, 1958

Kohon G: The Dead Mother: The Work of André Green. London, Routledge, 1999

Panksepp J, Biven L: The Archaeology of Mind. New York, Norton, 2012

Rey JH: Schizoid phenomena in the borderline, in Advances in the Psychotherapy of the Borderline Patient. Edited by LeBoit J, Cappari A. New York, Jason Aronson, 1979, pp 449–484

Rockland LH: Supportive Therapy for Borderline Patients: A Psychodynamic Approach. New York, Guilford, 1989

Rosenfeld H: Considerations regarding the psychoanalytic approach to acute and chronic schizophrenia. Int J Psychoanal 35:35–140, 1954

Rudolph G: Strukturbezogene Psychotherapie. Stuttgart, Germany, Schattauer, 2013

Searles HF: Collected Papers on Schizophrenia and Related Subjects. New York, International Universities Press, 1965

Spillius E, O'Shaughnessy E: Projective Identification: The Fate of a Concept. London, Routledge, 2012

Stone MH: Introductory comments on psychoanalytically oriented treatment of schizophrenia, in Treating Schizophrenic Patients: A Clinical Analytic Approach. Edited by Stone MH, Albert HD, Forrest DV, Arieti S. New York, McGraw Hill, 1983, pp 21–64

Stone MH: Exploratory psychotherapy in schizophrenia-spectrum patients: a reevaluation in the light of long-term follow-up of schizophrenic and borderline patients. Bull Menninger Clin 50:287–306, 1986

Wallerstein R: Forty-two Lives in Treatment: A Study of Psychotherapy and Psychoanalysis. New York, Guilford, 1986

Winnicott D: The Maturational Processes and the Facilitating Environment. New York, International Universities Press, 1965

Yeomans F, Clarkin JF, Kernberg OF: Transference Focused Psychotherapy for Borderline Personality Disorder: A Clinical Guide. Washington, DC, American Psychiatric Publishing, 2015

CHAPTER 5

Affective Dominance, Dyadic Relationship, and Mentalization

The main objective of this chapter is to highlight the two dominant frames within which therapists decide where and how to intervene with their interpretive efforts in the psychoanalytic treatment or psychoanalytic psychotherapy—specifically, transference-focused psychotherapy (TFP)—of severe personality disorders. These frames are 1) affective dominance and 2) the diagnosis of the corresponding dissociated or repressed internalized object relationship enacted in the transference.

Affective Dominance

When therapists approach a patient's communication within a psychotherapeutic session with an attitude of "evenly suspended attention" (Freud 1914/1958) or "without memory nor desire" (Bion 1967), multiple issues may emerge in rapid sequence in the patient's free associations, the accompanying nonverbal aspects of the patient's behavior, and an upsurge in the therapist's countertransference. Which of these various manifestations should be taken up first or which combination of these issues dominates are questions that therapists intuitively explore based on their impression of the affective dominance of the material. Identifying what is affectively dominant in the session corresponds to what Otto Fenichel (1941) called the economic, dynamic, and structural aspects of interpretation—namely, the dominant libidinal issue of the moment (the economic viewpoint), the interpretation of the defense against an underlying impulse and its respective motivation (the dynamic viewpoint), and the analysis of the placement of this unconscious intrapsychic conflict in terms of the relationship between superego, ego, and id (the structural viewpoint).

In contemporary psychoanalytic object relations theory, the clinical focus on predominant libidinal drive manifestations is complemented by the focus on aggressive ones, and the focus on drives is replaced by exploration of self- and object representations and their corresponding affects. The economic viewpoint of interpretation signals the dominant affective development at a certain point in the session. Affective dominance also relates to Bion's (1967) concept of the "selected fact" and, in more general terms, reflects an essential assumption of contemporary object relations theory that both defensive and impulsive manifestations of unconscious conflicts emerge as the activation of internalized units of object relations, in other words, a relation between self and object within the frame of a dominant affect. Affective dominance, in short, is the dominant internalized object relationship that emerges in response to its organizing affective experience and expression—the dominant desires or fears aroused by the intrapsychic conflict being activated.

Affective dominance can be evaluated by the therapist's simultaneous exploration of the content of free associations, the patient's accompanying nonverbal behavior, and the therapist's own countertransference. In standard psychoanalytic treatment, the development of affective dominance is more gradual than what typically evolves in psychoanalytic psychotherapy, particularly in TFP of patients with severe personality disorders. Patients with neurotic personality organization whose communications predominantly evolve through their free associations provide more time in which the therapist can orient him- or herself to what is dominant in those free associations and to what extent the nonverbal behaviors or countertransference overshadow them. Patients with neurotic personality organization usually can express their emotional reality through subjectively experienced, verbally communicated, and affectively invested thoughts, fantasies, memories, aspirations, desires, and fears. In contrast, patients with severe personality disorders have limited capacity for emotional cognitive communication through free association, and nonverbal behavior often dominates their interactions with the therapist from the beginning of treatment. The chaos that easily emerges in the psychotherapeutic sessions, such as rapid shifts of cognitive content; contradictory, eruptive behaviors; and powerful countertransference reactions, complicates the determination of what is affectively dominant. Thus, the focus on affective dominance is a natural aspect of the therapist's evenly suspended attention, and with neurotic patients, the decision of what to approach first is interpreted by the therapist primarily through the content of the patient's free associations.

There are also cases in standard psychoanalytic treatment in which nonverbal behavior acquires affective dominance, sometimes even at the beginning of treatment. For example, a patient with a narcissistic personality structure started his first analytic session by mentioning that he had had a dream in which he was in a room where everything was made of stone. The stone table, stone chairs, and stone pictures on the walls had reminded him of a painting by René Magritte with these characteristics. That corresponding painting by Magritte also immediately came to my mind. The patient went on to describe a door in the room, also made of stone, that he could open and look outside, where there was an enormous field covered with stones. "Only stones," he added with a clearly ironic tone and smile that conveyed pleasure. He then fell silent. I wondered what had come to his mind regarding that picture, and he repeated "just stones, stones, nothing else," in a tone that was now ironic and defiant.

I pointed out that the most significant reaction he seemed to have to this dream was a sense of pleasure about there being nothing but stones and that no other meaning could emerge from that experience. I wondered whether this implied a question in his mind as to what extent the search for unknown meanings in psychoanalytic technique really was a questionable enterprise. The patient immediately agreed; he said that he had been questioning whether psychoanalysis would really help him with his problems. He then became somewhat restless and wondered if I might be annoyed by his admission of doubt. I replied that it was important he express whatever came to his mind as openly as he could and that I sensed him doing just that, including experiencing a certain degree of satisfaction that no other meaning could be extracted from his dream about stones. Both his expression of doubt about being helped by psychoanalysis and his strange pleasure about the lack of meaning were interesting. This was the beginning of a long and complex analysis of his unconscious need to maintain a superior stance and of his unconscious fears of being dominated and humiliated by me as a sadistic parental object. Here, affective dominance emerged in a combination of verbal and nonverbal behavior to which was added a corresponding countertransference reaction on my part: I became slightly annoyed by his making fun of dream analysis.

The emergence of affective dominance tends to be much slower and subtle in the case of neurotic personality organization. For example, a patient with a hysterical personality disorder and significant sexual inhibition tended to pull down her dress repeatedly while she reclined on the couch, to a degree clearly beyond what would be needed to ensure no excessive exhibition of her legs. Meanwhile, she communicated important issues through free association regarding conflicts with her husband and her mother that were affectively dominant at that time. Only after months of treatment, in a session in which she had great difficulty carrying out free associations and communicating affectively meaningful content, did this particular gesture of straightening out her dress become affectively dominant—in other words, the most important issue occurring in the session. I suggested that she associate about her repetitive and exaggerated attempts at modesty, and she responded with a sequence of thoughts regarding her fear of my becoming sexually excited by her and her related fantasies of my seducing her and making her my sexual slave. Over several sessions, her fearfulness of male sexual aggression in the transference led to deeper levels of her oedipal conflicts. Her competitive behaviors in her relationship with her husband, which had dominated earlier in treatment, and her related deep fantasies and struggles to overcome her perceived inferiority as a woman had coincided with a defensive idealization of me that shifted into aggressive competitiveness. Her unconscious oedipal wishes to sexually seduce father emerged as the deeper impulse being defended against, represented by her dress-pulling behavior. It took a long time, weeks to months, for the affective dominance of that behavior to occupy a central attention of the session. In general, in the case of neurotic personality organization, dominant transference subjects emerge with clarity over a period of time by means of their acquiring, again and again, affective dominance.

In the case of severe personality disorders with a predominance of splitting mechanisms and related primitive defensive operations, the simultaneous emergence in consciousness of severely dissociated and contradictory conflictual themes during a session makes the evaluation of affective dominance more complex and urgent. The ability of these patients to communicate dominant unconscious conflicts through free association is much more limited; they express their dominant conflicts in both verbal and nonverbal behaviors, the intensity and invasive nature of which tend to generate rapidly intensifying countertransference reactions. These patients also often engage in destructive and self-destructive behavior, which intensifies the countertransference reaction and raises the question as to what extent the therapist's interpretive approach will be sufficient to avoid disastrous consequences for the patient's life. Thus, predominant attention to free association will not gradually clarify affective dominance by itself, and an urgent need may exist to decide how to intervene based on the combined analysis of verbal and nonverbal communication and countertransference.

For example, a young woman with a histrionic infantile personality disorder presented with severe daily conflicts with her mother and failure in her college studies. The patient began a session by briefly mentioning how tired she was because of the intense work in preparing for a forthcoming examination at school. She rapidly shifted into relating a fight with her boyfriend that eventually involved her mother criticizing her for her treatment of that relationship. An intense emotional, detailed commentary on the latest affect storm with her mother ensued. She suspected me of being on her boyfriend's side of the issue they were arguing and expressed distrust as to whether I also agreed with her mother. At the same time, I was struggling in my own mind with a concern over her forthcoming examination, which I knew would be crucial in determining whether she would pass the year or fail. We both knew that if she failed she would have to leave school, because her paid fellowship was conditioned on her not failing any of the school years.

The patient was almost yelling as she described her mother's impossible behavior, while I became increasingly anxious about the danger to her fellowship, which, at that moment, seemed to be outside of her emotional awareness. I decided to ignore the affect storm about her mother and to interpret her lack of concern over the threat to her academic career as the main issue affecting her. I pointed out that she was using her mother's behavior as a defense against her unconscious temptation to fail the year and be expelled from school. Despite her yelling attacks toward her mother, I made my point loud enough to be heard and to make her hesitantly pay attention and become anxious. Obviously, many other aspects of this patient's life and behavior warranted this interpretation on my part, but the formulation of this issue at that particular moment came from my assessing it as affectively dominant based on my own intense countertransference reaction.

Most therapeutic decisions regarding affective dominance and the interpretive interventions derived from that judgment are less dramatic and urgent. I selected this one because it also highlights the problem of countertransference features fostering the decision about affective dominance. To what extent should countertransference reactions be used in this way, and to what extent might they reflect countertransference acting out being expressed as interpretive priorities? An ongoing task of the therapist treating severe personality disorders is to obtain a realistic assessment of urgencies in the patient's life by analyzing the therapeutic situation in the time between sessions to protect from making sudden judgments during sessions that may indeed reflect countertransference acting out. Making an overall assessment of therapeutic urgencies as a general judgment about the patient provides a frame against which intense countertransference reactions may guide decisions regarding what is affectively dominant. A realistic common-sense awareness of the patient's total life situation—the areas of work and profession, love and sex, social life and creativity—provides a sense that one's openness or potential countertransference disposition can be trusted in the next session and can acquire the security of interpretive intervention based on what develops within the session itself.

Sometimes, a casual reference to a subject in the middle of free associations focused on a completely different area conveys to the therapist a sense that something strange yet meaningful has emerged and then disappeared from the patient's conscious awareness within seconds. This may lead the therapist to focus on something imperative that clearly needs to be understood. Drawing the patient's attention to the dissonant element in his or her communication may reveal an affectively dominant issue, what Bion (1967) calls an "accretion" or super-condensation of meaning.

The assumption of a "normal" therapeutic relationship as a precondition for both psychoanalysis and TFP (which technically comes closest to psychoanalysis) implies, in Loewald's (1960) description, a relationship between a realistically dependent patient who needs to be helped and who trusts the therapist's knowledge, interest, concerned disposition, and expertise—without expecting the therapist to be omniscient or omnipotent—and a therapist who has the adequate knowledge, commitment, and concern for the patient to be of help. Transference developments may be diagnosed and interpreted as deviations from the "normal" therapeutic relationship that appear within the patient's material and interactions with the analyst. In the course of standard psychoanalysis, the patient on the couch and the therapist sitting behind the patient formally confirm the assumed normal relationship, although, in the course of treatment, significant shifts in the patient's attitude signal the developments of the transference. This process develops gradually, and the example of the patient who dreamed about stones reflects an unusually early dominance of the transference. In the psychoanalytic psychotherapy of severe personality disorders, seen in face-to-face arrangements, rapid shifts from the assumed "normal" expected therapeutic relationship between patient and therapist may occur much more frequently. In fact, the more severe the patient's psychopathology, the earlier significant developments of the transference will distort that optimal relationship. Very often, in the absence of any reasonable attitude of collaboration from patients with severe character pathology, the therapist may need to establish a sufficiently secure therapeutic frame to permit the treatment to proceed. The therapeutic alliance between therapist and patient under these conditions may be practically zero at the start of the treatment, and only systematic analysis of negative transferences may gradually establish a degree of collaboration between them.

Under these conditions, what is affectively dominant usually implies the transference from the very start. However, with such severely ill patients, mutually dissociated, split-off transference developments emerge and alternate rapidly from negative to positive and back to negative affective dominance in the respective activation of dissociative internalized object relations. Splitting and projective mechanisms produce rapidly shifting representations of self and other, so that at any given moment patients may believe themselves to be the helpless victim of an uncaring, callous therapist, only to oscillate to a position of superiority over a devalued, useless therapist within the same session. The problem, then, is to determine relatively rapidly what aspect of this dissociated transference represents affective dominance at that point.

A woman in her middle twenties with schizoid personality disorder who worked as an advanced student in a mental health service complained bitterly over the hypocrisy of one of her supervisors, who had treated a patient as though she were very concerned about and interested in her when, in fact, the supervisor was mostly concerned that the patient obey the rules and not cause problems. The patient told me this with a rigid, cold, and resentful attitude and then fell silent. I had the fantasy that she expected me now to say that she may have a similar experience of me as someone who pretended to be interested in her, but I saw this as provocation for me to do the obvious, so I also remained silent, wondering what was really going on.

In the middle of this silence, the patient looked at a huge picture of Vienna in the 16th century that was hanging in my office and said, in a slightly ironic tone, "Here you have a picture of the city where you lived as a child, who threw you out, and now you are longing for them." That comment came totally unexpected and immediately touched very personal issues relating to my relationship with Vienna, the city of my childhood. I sensed a mixture of an ironic attitude of superiority, which I had detected before, and a sense of the patient's honest empathy with what she saw as an internal conflict with mother projected onto me. It took me a while to react, and then I said, "It is difficult to deal with a combination of rage and longing about being abandoned by the most important person in one's life."

This illustrates several internalized object relations emerging simultaneously: 1) the patient's identification with a dominant, ironic mother rejecting her child, with the child experiencing mother as offering phony concern; 2) the alternative projection onto me of mother and of herself as rejected child, and 3) the apparent dominant affect directed towards her supervisor at work. I decided that the relationship with me was affectively dominant, and there were significant connections between the various aspects of the overall difficulty in the relationship with the internal mother image of this patient.

The significant difference between the protective structure provided by the couch in standard psychoanalysis and the face-to-face position in psychoanalytic psychotherapy has received surprising confirmation in the shared observation I have had with colleagues who, like myself, have been carrying out psychoanalytic treatment online using Zoom as our medium. Patients in psychoanalytic treatment receiving three to five sessions a week typically spend extended time not looking at the analyst in the Zoom image but appearing to concentrate on themselves as they carry out free association; however, when dominant feelings toward the analyst emerge, their face-to-face contact is intense and rapidly shifting. On the other hand, we have found that patients with borderline personality disorder maintain fairly regular eye contact. This illustrates the different structure of standard psychoanalysis, which fosters analytic focus on the communication of subjective experience via free associations as the dominant channel of information, from the face-to-face setting of psychoanalytic psychotherapy, which tolerates and fosters nonverbal communication through behavioral shifts in the session. This is a challenge and an advantage of psychoanalytic psychotherapy because it demands fast decision-making regarding affective dominance but facilitates earlier assessment of dominant characterological defenses that emerge as transference resistances.

In psychoanalysis, the therapist is focused primarily on the content of free association and maintains an empathic attitude toward the emotional significance of the patient's discourse. The therapist's attitude, we might say, is dominated by his or her introjective identification with the patient's subjective experience. With patients in TFP, despite an equally important emphasis on free associations, the combination of face-to-face encounters and the severity of the psychopathology privileges the expression of unconscious intrapsychic conflicts through behavior. Thus, rather than having only the emotional content of free association, therapists are confronted with actual and frequently urgent information expressed in their patient's behavior from the very beginning of treatment. For patients with severe personality disorders in TFP, therapists' attention is rapidly focused on the behavioral distortions that shift the patient–therapist relationship away from the optimal "normal" defined at the beginning of the treatment. Therapists tend to focus mostly on projective identifications from patients that register in their countertransference. Thus, a different empathic focus is determined by standard psychoanalytic technique compared with the psychoanalytic psychotherapy represented by TFP. The fact that transference becomes an important source of information from the outset of treatment does not mean, however, that it always constitutes what is affectively dominant at any given point. Although transference developments most frequently determine what is affectively dominant, the therapist carrying out standard psychoanalytic technique or TFP must be open to affectively dominant information related to events outside the sessions that is communicated verbally and nonverbally and sometimes also through countertransference. There are, in short, clinically varying roots to the rapid assessment of what is affectively dominant at any point of the sessions. These can be interpreted through a combined analysis of verbal and nonverbal communication, countertransference, and potentially ominous developments in external reality that are being successfully split from entering the material of the session.

One situation in which the assessment of affective dominance becomes particularly acute and crucial is the analytic exploration of sessions that include extended periods of silence. Long periods of silence may be the result of multiple transference developments, such as patients with oppositional behavior under conditions of predominantly strong negative transferences, whatever the origin; patients with schizoid personalities who have regressed to the earliest stages of internalized object relations development, where only behavioral manifestations reflect their early traumatization and cognitive/affective memory structures are absent; patients with paranoid personalities and intense persecutory panic; or patients with severe depression who devastatingly self-devalue everything that comes to their mind as useless or malignant. We developed a technical approach in TFP to deal with this situation; we stimulate the silent patient after a few minutes—"You remain silent"—and then wait for the patient's reaction. Meanwhile, we assess the shift in the emotional relation between patient and therapist that occurs in response to that stimulation. After a few minutes, we interpret to the patient the potentially significant shift in his or her emotional involvement that has occurred during the past few minutes. Then we wait a few more minutes while observing the new shifts in how the patient's reaction to this interpretation manifests. If silence continues, we again stimulate the patient to say what is on his or her mind and then follow the same sequence of waiting and observing.

It is usually not difficult to solve long silences by gradually interpreting their shifting transference meanings, although at times it may take a few sessions to fully resolve this particular resistance. This interpretive work focuses intensively on manifestations of affective developments in the patient, as reflected in facial expression and dissociated general movements, and on countertransference reactions—the therapist's fantasied development of reasons for the patient's silence and the associations that may evolve, stimulated by the simultaneous intense presence of a silent patient and a silent therapist in a momentarily mysterious interaction.

I have found that, at times, extended silences thus explored unexpectedly illuminate major issues in the treatment, particularly the development of transferences that have been present, yet ignored—intuitively captured and yet not previously formulated by the therapist. One patient began the session relating a chaotic dream to which I stimulated him to associate, which brought about more trivial details that took time to explain and did not lead to any further understanding. He presented all of this in a monotonous, mechanical way that had a hypnotic effect on me, and I had to struggle to remain awake. The patient finally looked at me without any particular expression in his face and fell silent. I had no comment to make about the dream, except that it seemed confusing and that thinking about it seemed to lead him into more confusion or expression of trivialities. He nodded, continuing in silence but now scrutinizing me very actively. I was struggling with the sense of fatigue when the patient suddenly said, "You're falling asleep." Now it was my turn to nod agreement and to look attentively at the patient (I was fully alert by now). The patient continued silent, looking at me with a slightly triumphant expression. After a few more minutes, I said "I think something in you has been trying to convince me that nothing important is going on in you; that, in effect, you do not have an internal life that relates you to anybody else and that you are not different from me, who pretends to be interested in another person, namely in you, when in reality I am totally indifferent, falling asleep because of the meaningless of this encounter. And I have a sense that something in you felt triumphant with your assessment of this situation, in which neither you nor I are alive." Several minutes of silence followed, while I sensed that things were going on within the patient. He finally said, "I've been thinking about what you said, and I can't tell whether it's very true or whether it's one of these fancy explanations that psychoanalysts indulge in," to which I responded, "I believe you are divided between one part of you that would wish me to be dead—feeling relieved that it's not only you who feels that you are dead—and another part of you that would want me to remain alive and interested in you in spite of your efforts to eliminate both of us. But the fact that I can remain alive to try to understand what is going on generates resentment in you, and you obtain no relief from my continuing to be alive with you." By this time, we were both wide awake, and the patient said he felt relieved.

Affective dominance may lie in the patient's subjective experience, for example, in the case of a patient who presents himself in the session by letting us know that he has just been diagnosed with a severe, potentially life-threatening illness. A realistic anxiety dominates the patient's experience and, as we learn about it, our own emotional reaction as well. There is no question here what issue is the most important to take up. At times, the intensity of the patient's affective reaction, an affect storm, clearly dominates the session and requires analytic effort to both keep its behavioral communication within certain limits and to provide a cognitive-emotional frame—a containment of it—that, by clarifying its function within the patient's dominant conflict, explores its deeper significance and sources. At times, affective dominance clearly derives from a countertransference reaction in the therapist, and here it is important to clarify the extent to which this is an acute reaction relating to this particular session, to be understood in terms of the patient's unconscious intrapsychic conflict now being enacted, and to what extent the therapist's deeper transference dispositions may be contributing to the powerful affective development of the countertransference. This is different from chronic countertransference developments that may distort the therapist's technically neutral position and interfere with the therapeutic freedom to listen "without memory nor desire." Chronic countertransference reactions, signaled by a permanent shift in the therapist's internal relation to a particular patient over a period of time, must be explored and resolved outside the treatment sessions by the therapist's own self-analysis or consultation with a colleague; when resolved, they may contribute important new understanding of transference developments that previously had been experienced but not understood by the therapist.

Barranger and Barranger (1966) described "bastions," unconscious collusions between patients and analysts in which certain subjects are not touched. These require a careful, long-range exploration of what the initial objectives of the treatment were and to what extent those objectives have somewhere been restricted, out of the patient's unconscious resistances to resolve a problem that generates enormous anxiety and the therapist's unconscious "contamination" by the patient's fearfulness over exploring this issue. Two major therapeutic contributions may prevent, diagnose, or resolve such a situation. The first of these is a careful exploration at the beginning of the treatment of the symptoms, difficulties, problems, and expectations that limit the patient's gratifying and effective life and the extent to which the patient's objectives correspond or are in harmony with those of the therapist. This initial knowledge may constitute an important alerting system to issues that, although important at the beginning of the treatment, seem to have disappeared in the course of therapeutic developments. Second, the therapist must use his or her own life experience to make a mature assessment of ordinary human relationships and the tasks and difficulties of work and profession, love and sex, and social life and creativity.

Sometimes it is only the therapist's mature level of practical common sense that, combined with the knowledge of the patient's initial reasons for treatment, facilitates awareness of a mutual collusion in avoiding significant conflicts that are interfering with the patient's life situation. This discovery of areas of collusion may evoke a powerful affective response in the therapist, who—by what may be called a meta-psychological process—becomes alerted to a major difficulty the patient is avoiding and dares to include it in the therapeutic dialogue. Here, affective dominance is linked to the therapist's overall evaluation of the patient's restricted status and conduct in life, the patient's lack of full development of his or her potential, and the need to explore these issues, in contrast to the potential collusion with the patient in avoiding them. This kind of situation emerges rarely in cases of standard psychoanalytic technique, in which the patient's integrated identity usually is reflected in reasonable life goals and an awareness of conflicts regarding them. In the case of patients with severe personality disorders, such unconscious collusions are not uncommon. These patients' severe failure in some areas of life, emptiness regarding love relations, struggles or failures in the workplace, or specific difficulties in life arrangements are so severe that they tend to obscure other areas of conflict avoidance that emerge in the treatment. Thus, affective dominance sometimes derives from a gradual process of evaluation and commitment to the patient. Such developments will reflect healthy "disturbances" emerging in affective dominance derived from the therapist's concerns.

In conclusion, affective dominance determines the interpretive interventions to be made at each point of the sessions that warrant interpretive action. It permits diagnosis of the dominant internalized object relationships, which are the building blocks of the dyadic and triadic object relations that constitute psychic experiences in normality and pathology, the fundamental target of psychoanalytic interventions. It leads to the emergence of an aspect of the patient's self relating to a specific internalized object, and the enactment of the relation between the self and object in the transference. Affective dominance leads to the dominant relationship between patient and therapist.

Present Dyadic Relationship and Mentalization

Affective dominance and the related self and object relationship are the predominant concerns of the therapist practicing standard psychoanalysis or TFP across the spectrum of severity of personality disorders. I refer to the practical concern emerging in every session that orients the therapist toward the predominant internalized object relationship being activated at any point during that session. The dominant internalized object relationship, reflecting defensive or impulsive aspects of repressed or dissociated unconscious conflicts involving aggressive and libidinal impulses, also emerges as the salient issue in the transference and is the primary object of transference interpretation. This dominant object relationship, which emerges in the patient's material through free association, nonverbal communication, countertransference activation, or even a threatening development in the patient's external reality, must be diagnosed, whether it seems to involve a conflict of the patient outside the sessions or directly as a transference development. Practically, dominant conflicts outside the treatment sessions either reflect displaced aspects of present transference developments or, eventually, will evolve into transference issues in the course of their exploration. The evaluation of affective dominance is the first task of the psychotherapist in psychoanalytic modalities of treatment, and the evaluation of the underlying activated internalized object relationship is a second, closely related task. An internalized object relation involves an essentially dyadic interaction between self and other, linked by the affect in which it was embedded and enacted in the transference (Caligor et al. 2018; Kernberg 2020).

A college student with serious inhibition, failure in his studies despite high intelligence, chronic difficulties with other classmates and friends, and ongoing alternation between excessive fear and rebellious behavior toward authorities began a session complaining about the inadequate ways in which a professor had explained the material that had to be prepared for a written examination. He also complained about the lack of collaboration to be expected from a friend and classmate, the poor scheduling and coordination of tasks expected by the school, and the lack of understanding by his mother of the hardships he was experiencing at school. He talked with resentment about how these people were failing him, but in a monotonous voice, as though he were reciting all his troubles without really expecting the therapist to be of help and feeling rather irritated about complaining to a useless source of understanding. The monotony and the hopelessness of his complaints combined to create an atmosphere of demandingness and, at the same time, to convey his conviction that nothing in this session would be of help. The combination of these features reflected in his monotonous discourse also conveyed a sense of tiredness and distance. Reflecting on my own experiences, I felt I was not really available to him emotionally at this point. I ventured the suggestion that I was experiencing him as a very frustrated, demanding child who is angrily but also hopelessly making inordinate demands on a mother—me—who pretends to be interested but truly is indifferent and does not want to be bothered, intensifying his resentment and hopelessness. As we explored the patient's reactions to this interpretation, he confirmed his view of me as distant, sleepy, and feigning interest and expressed the intense frustration he was feeling because of all the pressure he was under. He wished to let it all go and to dedicate himself to enjoying video games.

With further exploration of the patient's experience of himself and of me, the monotony of his discourse shifted into an intense, angry discourse. I, in turn, became fully emotionally involved and interested in this particular object relationship. Thus, a momentary change in the atmosphere of the session emerged. However, toward the middle of the session, the affective tone shifted again as the patient seemingly lost interest and became distracted by his plan to buy some electronic equipment. His associations became fully involved in a detailed comparison of alternative electronic instruments. My efforts to return to the issue we were discussing led nowhere. I suggested through various interventions that he seemed to be moving away from examining what was going on in the session, but although he responded politely to my comment, it was with clear impatience with my attempts to direct his attention from his shopping concerns. I began to feel that I was trying to obtain his attention, as if it were attention to me and my emotional needs, while the patient acted with a distancing indifference and with irritation at my interference with his preferred topic. Before the end of the session, I was able to point out to the patient that the relationship between a demanding, frustrated child and an indifferent, distancing mother had been replicated between us, but now with role reversals: I was now in the role of the demanding child wanting attention, while he was in the role of his indifferent, aloof mother.

This short summary illustrates the effort to diagnose the predominant internalized object relationship enacted in the transference: the patient's frustrated and demanding aspect of his infantile self and the corresponding indifferent and rejecting aspect of his mother. This relationship was enacted and then reenacted with role reversal that would permit the patient, through interpretation of this repetitive activation, to become aware of the importance of that unresolved conflict in his mind and in his present relationship with me. As part of this process, he became aware of and resolved his unconscious identification with both self and object in this activated dyadic relationship. This relationship was an important component of his tendency to abandon his studies and finding them to be an imposition, his resentment of the teachers' perceived lack of interest and concern, and his provocative efforts to obtain a particular professor's attention that were being undermined by the irritation he was causing. All these various aspects of the patient's difficulties at school were now represented in the activation of this particular object relationship, which I was able to help the patient realize was in fact a distortion of reality. It gradually became clear to him that the teacher was neither as rejecting nor as demanding as the patient perceived and that his own behavior had provoked the professor to react to him in an irritated and sometimes rejecting way.

At the same time, the patient was aware that I was interested in him and that, by his coming to the sessions, carrying out free associations, and being open to an exchange with me, a reality of a cooperative relationship was evolving that corresponded to my role, the patient's role, his interest in getting help and learning in the treatment, and my concerned efforts to help him know himself and the nature of his difficulties. In other words, as I helped the patient become fully aware of the unconscious relationship activated in the transference, I also helped him become aware that another, more realistic relationship was developing that permitted us to understand the troublesome dissociated relationship that reflected his unresolved unconscious conflict from the past. The trigger for exploring this particular relationship was my sense that this issue was affectively dominant at the beginning of the session, rather than the subject matter of his associations—the various aspects of the professor's behavior, his classmate's unavailability, and so on. The affective dominance of the interaction between us in the transference led to the possibility of fully exploring the enacted internalized object relationship.

One may describe the initial aspect of my interpretive intervention as an effort to increase the patient's awareness of his feelings toward me, of what he perceived as my attitude toward him, and of the reality of the interaction: his monotonous recitation of issues of his daily life and my forced interest and underlying boredom. This may be described as an effort to increase his mentalization—that is, his awareness of his intentionality in his emotional experience and of the intentionality in my emotional experience. Gradually, we were able to clarify the difference between this awareness of our interactions at that level, on the one hand, and our parallel implicit interactions reflecting the agreed-upon structure of the treatment—that is, our respective collaborative tasks for each other. I was, in fact, contributing to his mentalization at the level of the activated fantasy structure that I interpreted and at the level of interaction in reality. One might say that a double, parallel mentalization was gradually achieved.

However, in contrast to a treatment approach that would help the patient become aware of the unrealistic conflictual aspect of the activated object relationship in the transference and of the realistic nature of our relationship (rather than letting it be distorted by this enactment of the pathological one), my intention was to preserve the full presence of that activated conflictual object relationship, including role reversals in it, with the expectation that the pathological relationship potentially was serving a defensive function against an alternative relationship that was not yet available. Rather than "normalizing" our relationship by mentalizing the reality aspects of our interaction, I tried to preserve the experience of the transference regression to analyze its defensive function against an assumed opposite one that reflected the "impulsive" side of the unconscious conflict. In the case of this patient, this "opposite" was an idealized relationship in which he would be able to depend on me completely as someone who was lovingly dedicated to him. In this idealized relationship, I would become an ideal parental figure who combined the features of both parents and reflected an intense, dependent, sexualized attachment to his father, which served as a displacement from his insecure attachment to his mother and a sexualized negative oedipal conflict. This patient indeed presented strong homosexual impulses and bisexual behaviors linked to this alternative but presently not available internalized object relationship, against which the relationship that was dominantly enacted in the session served a defensive function.

In more general terms, although a certain activated transference disposition may serve a defensive function against a deeper repressed one, as is typical for neurotic structures with well-integrated identity formation, in the case of borderline personality organization, the desired relationship representing the deeper level of the conflict usually is not repressed but, rather, is dissociated. Splitting defenses separate alternative, contradictory behavior patterns that superficially may impress one as chaotic character traits and only are discovered in their implicit defense/impulse structure as part of transference analysis.

An important difference in the activation of internalized object relationships in the case of patients with neurotic personality organization and borderline personality organization—in other words, between the healthier spectrum of personality disorders and the severe degrees of personality disorders—resides in the relative stability of the self-concept that has been integrated as part of one's identity in neurotic personality organization compared with the dissociated, split concepts of self and others in borderline personality organization. This is an important, practical clinical difference. Patients with neurotic personality organization usually reflect different levels of unconscious conflicts in terms of activation of the corresponding internalized object relations in the transference, but without the high frequency of interchange between self and object enactment and projection as in borderline personality organization. The patient usually enacts aspects of his or her infantile self, and the therapist enacts various objects of the patient's infancy and childhood.

Although the corresponding technical instruments are basically the same as in standard psychoanalysis—that is, interpretation, transference analysis, technical neutrality, and countertransference utilization, TFP is based on the strategy of interpreting mutually dissociated idealized and persecutory internalized object relationships in the transference. It follows a sequence of identifying corresponding self- and object representations in the interaction as framed by the corresponding dominant affect, followed by analysis of their enactments and projections within the transference. This may be construed as "who is doing what to whom." Clarifying the internalized object relations, interpreting their alternative enactments and projections, and interpreting the mutually dissociated idealized and persecutory object relationship thus constitute the essential strategy of TFP.

It is of interest to compare TFP with mentalization-based therapy (MBT) for borderline conditions. MBT has also been expanded to treat patients across a range of severe personality disorders in general (Fonagy et al. 2002) and attempts to help patients acquire a more realistic awareness of the mental states they enact and the states expressed by others with whom they relate, particularly the therapist, so that they acquire a more realistic awareness of the emotional significance of their own experience, expression, and intentionality and of those of the therapist. Patients are helped to acquire, through identification with the therapist's interest and capability to empathize with their emotional experience, the capacity to do the same in their interactions with significant others. MBT thus explores the nature of the self- and object representations enacted by patients and helps them gradually transform their distorted perceptions into more realistic perceptions of self and other in the therapeutic interaction, leading to improved understanding of intentions, communication, and mutual responsiveness. MBT is an effective way for correcting the distortions of patients' perceptions of self and other in intimate interactions and permits the improvement in patients' functioning by increasing their capacity for self-reflection and the realistic assessment of their actual relationships.

By comparison, the initial stages of TFP are quite similar to MBT in the therapist's efforts to clarify the nature of the experience of self- and object representations activated in the transference, but TFP differs significantly in its efforts not to reduce, normalize, or eliminate that experience but rather to maintain and investigate it in a parallel exploration of the more realistic aspects of the relationship between patient and therapist. The attempt to clarify yet maintain interest in the nature of the enacted pathological relationship facilitates the gradual integration of contradictory internalized object relationships and permits patients to acquire a more realistic awareness of self and of others by overcoming the original split between idealized and persecutory affect states. Thus, the split internalized object relationship eventually becomes unified and facilitates an integration of identity that permits, in turn, realistic evaluation of self and others in all relationships, beginning with the strengthening of the "normal" aspects of the therapeutic relationship. The purpose of TFP is a radical normalization of the personality structure, an effort to integrate the patient's capacity for a full, effective, and satisfactory experience in work and profession, love and sex, and social life and creativity. It is based on a systematic interpretation of the transference rather than an attempt to normalize transference-determined behavior as in MBT, which focuses on the development of more realistic awareness of emotional motivation and intentionality of self and others, their expression, assessment, and regulation.

In TFP, the concept of mentalization is used to differentiate two major stages of the development of a realistic assessment of motivation of self and others, represented, respectively, by identity diffusion and normal identity. Within this conception, a first stage of development, covering roughly the first 2 or 3 years of life, is characterized by distinct, mutually split-off, idealized, and persecutory segments of experience that are dominated by positive or negative affect systems and the internalized object relations associated with them. Here *mentalization* refers to the capacity to realistically assess one's present state of mind, intentionality, and view of self and other within the present affective state linking them, with no connection to alternative ways of experiencing self or others at different moments of affect activation. Self-reflection is limited to the presently dominant affective state. In contrast, in a second stage of development, when mentalization reaches *maturity*, the activation of any particular affective state and the self-reflection connected with it automatically implies a capacity to locate that particular state within the general experience of the total personality of self and a comparison between the current moment and the general approach to self and others in reality that is derived from the total dynamic integration of all internalized object relations. In TFP, we use this specific way of referring to two stages of mentalization rather than the more general concept of emotional introspection or insight as a nonspecific, general self-reflectiveness that naturally develops with life experience, including both peak affect states and the development of cognitive knowledge at times of low affect activation.

References

Barranger M, Barranger W: Insight and the analytic situation, in Psychoanalysis in the Americas. Edited by Litman R. New York, International Universities Press, 1966, pp 56–72

Bion W: Second Thoughts: Selected Papers on Psychoanalysis. London, Heinemann, 1967

Caligor E, Kernberg OF, Clarkin JF, Yeomans FE: Psychodynamic Therapy for Personality Pathology: Treating Self and Interpersonal Functioning. Washington, DC, American Psychiatric Association Publishing, 2018

Fenichel O: Problems of Psychoanalytic Technique, Albany, NY, Psychoanalytic Quarterly Press, 1941

Fonagy P, Gergely G, Jurist EL, Target M: Affect Regulation, Mentalization and the Development of the Self. New York, Other Press, 2002

Freud S: Remembering, repeating, and working through (further recommendations on the technique of psycho-analysis II) (1914), in The Standard Edition of the Complete Psychological Works of Sigmund Freud, Vol 12. Translated and edited by Strachey J. 1958, pp 145–156

Kernberg OF: Object Relations Theory and Transference Analysis. Unpublished manuscript, 2020

Loewald H: On the therapeutic action of psycho-analysis. Int J Psychoanal 41:16–33, 1960

CHAPTER 6

Reflections on Supervision

The tasks of a supervisor of psychodynamic therapies may include the supervision of psychoanalysis by candidates in training, senior analysts interested in new approaches to technique, as well as therapists who are learning, at different levels of experience, to carry out psychoanalytically oriented psychotherapies. These psychotherapies include a broad range of treatment approaches: supportive psychotherapy based on psychoanalytic theory, transference-focused psychotherapy, mentalization-based psychotherapy, self-psychology, and others. Ideally, a psychodynamically oriented psychotherapist should be able to carry out several of these modalities of psychoanalytically based treatments.

Practically, specialization within this broad spectrum of application of psychoanalytic theory and technique is unavoidable, and the major focus of the corresponding literature has been on the supervision of psychoanalytic candidates, on the one hand, and of psychoanalytically oriented psychotherapists in a broad, rather nonspecific way, on the other

Published in *The American Journal of Psychoanalysis*, 79(3):265–283, 2019. Copyright © 2019 Association for the Advancement of Psychoanalysis. Reprinted with permission.

(Blomfield 1985). A challenge may arise when supervisor and supervisee are approaching a case from different schools of thought and modality, but each stands to learn from such an endeavor. This complexity, naturally, is enormously simplified when both supervisor and supervisee are part of the same educational or professional system—for example, from the same training institute—which should provide clearer boundaries around the tasks of both supervisor and supervisee. When a senior psychoanalyst supervises an independent practitioner in private practice, the expectations and responsibilities of both have to be negotiated much more carefully.

Regardless of whatever issues may arise from differences of setting (institutional or private), or theoretical underpinnings, clarifying mutual expectations and responsibilities in a supervisory enterprise applies to all cases. Therefore, a full discussion of the backgrounds, experiences, and expectations of both the supervisee and the supervisor is part of the process. Agreement about the joint task, based on a mutual understanding, should then lead to the choice of material best suited to the particular supervision (Kernberg 2010). Potentially problematic is disagreement over whether the supervisee needs to perform a careful diagnostic evaluation of the patient. The extent to which such a diagnostic evaluation is considered necessary or helpful varies enormously within different psychoanalytic orientations and depends, at least in part, on whether the supervisee is part of an academic institution or a private practitioner.

The responsibility for the treatment of the patient needs to be clarified. Ideally it should rest totally in the hands of the treating therapist, but if the therapist is part of a training institution, the supervisor may be involved in the responsibility for the patient as well, and that needs to be clarified. The supervisor should be responsible only for the supervision of the supervisee, and the supervisee should be either responsible for the treatment of the patient or responsible to an administrative superior within the institution in which the treatment takes place. Because ambiguity of this understanding may have legal consequences, and other administrative or educational issues may be involved, total clarity of these responsibilities is indispensable.

The next issue to consider is the purpose of the supervision and whether it is simply to improve learning and strengthen the supervisee's professional skills or whether it will include an evaluative function that affects the supervisee's advancement or standing within a training institute. If the supervision is part of an institutional training program, such as a psychoanalytic institute, this evaluation becomes an essential aspect of the supervisory process. The supervisor is both teacher and evaluator and has to live with this double function. This implies not only the supervisor's capacity to make a fair and objective evaluation of the supervisee's progress but also, very essentially, his or her capacity to convey to the supervisee honest conclusions about the supervisee's performance and progress. Under optimal circumstances, it will be a pleasurable process to congratulate the supervisee for his learning and progress and, to the contrary but, of course, painful to have to communicate to him that this supervisory process has not been working. Ideally, if a supervisory process fails, it may be preferable to interrupt it, consider it inconclusive, or offer the supervisee alternative supervisory possibilities so that the institutional evaluation of the supervisee can be arrived at by multiple sources of input (Tuckett 2005).

Having agreed upon the material to be presented in the supervisory sessions: communications by the patient, both verbal and nonverbal, and the therapist's reaction to the patient's presence and material—in other words, transference and countertransference developments in the course of the therapy sessions—as well as the dominant issues, conflicts, and themes to be analytically explored, a delicate task follows. An element of trust is required on the part of the supervisee to openly explore his reactions, fears, and fantasies about his patient, and in processing the tactful evaluation on the part of the supervisor. A relational process develops in the supervisory situation as well, which will be part of the responsibility of the supervisor to utilize in the context of this particular supervisory process (Greenberg 1997; Yerushalmi 2019).

The supervisor should freely share with the supervisee his own emotional reaction to the patient's material and the way the therapist is presenting it. This invites discussion of the therapist's countertransference reactions and expands the depth of the therapist's analysis of the transference/countertransference developments in sessions. This, under optimal circumstances, will increase openness and the potentially intimate nature of the supervisory process. In group supervision the process would be much more restricted. Using group processes to study individual responses to therapeutic material presented by a group member would probably elicit unique responses from each member. However, these often correspond to important, but possibly divergent, implications of the patient's and therapist's communications and may be useful to look at when analyzing transference/countertransference issues in the case under discussion.

Now comes the crucial question, what is the most important issue in the session that has just been examined? In other words, what seems to be affectively dominant among all aspects of verbal and nonverbal content, transference implications and countertransference reactions, and the potential influence of the patient's external reality? And if such a focus can be established, what does the therapist see as the potential conflictual aspect of this focus, what is surface and what is the defended-against impulse, the hypothetical unconscious meaning of the corresponding conflict? And beyond that immediate presentation of a determined conflict, how is it played out in terms of internal structures of the patient's personality? Is there a conflict between ego and superego, or between mutually split off aspects of the patient's self, potentially embedded in conflictual character traits (Kernberg 2018)?

This complex formulation, implicitly involving the supervisor's automatically exploring the material in the light of his general theory of technique and then focusing specifically on the presently dominating issues, constitutes the general frame of the supervisor's task. Formulating the economic (affective), dynamic (defense and impulse), structural (tripartite structure) aspects of the clinical material is, naturally, a metapsychological formulation that does not need to be involved in the simple diagnosis of what is going on in the "here and now" of a given session. As a general approach, the supervisor should have a full understanding of how the therapist is processing and understanding the patient's material before suggesting what he (the supervisor) might do based upon his internal model of understanding the nature of the material presented by the supervisee. It is important that the therapist be encouraged to convey his way of reasoning that would lead him to formulate a particular intervention. Supervision thus becomes the gradual communication, by the supervisor to the supervisee, of the supervisor's internal structure of organization of the material in terms of his personal theory of psychoanalytic technique, but only in response and reaction to the therapist's views.

The objective that the therapist should learn to integrate his discrete reactions to the supervisory material into a fully developed internal theory of psychoanalytic and psychodynamic principles that can be applied to a broad spectrum of interventions seems to be an important aspect of optimal supervision (Kernberg 2010). It does not mean that the supervisor should not react spontaneously, intuitively, rapidly, to what the supervisee is presenting to him, but, to the contrary, the supervisor should be able to rely on his emotional reaction and associations to the supervisory material in a way that would lead to a therapeutic intervention that forms part of a harmonic integration of his technical knowledge. That implies, if the supervisor carries out exclusively psychoanalytic supervision, a linkage with his particular psychoanalytic orientation and may make it relatively easy to convey his reasoning to the supervisee, as it overlaps with the supervisee's training in the same institution.

If supervisor and supervisee belong to different psychoanalytic institutions, with different "political" orientations, such differences can be ventilated and explored with openness and respect for the candidate's different "ideological" background. For a supervisor who is versed in "standard" psychoanalytical technique as well as in one or several alternative forms of psychoanalytical psychotherapy, such an integration may be a more complex process but, at the same time, offers the possibility of an integration in depth that may enrich his total knowledge, repertoire of interventions, and technical skills to deal with the unexpected developments in every treatment. And, of course, it permits the supervisor to supervise and treat a broad spectrum of patients, including the severe personality disorders and extreme self-destructive pathologies that often cannot be handled by a standard psychoanalytic approach. A supervisor's knowledge and experience about a broad spectrum of psychoanalytic psychotherapies also sharpens his capacity for exploring the nonverbal, behavioral aspects of the emotional elements of patients' presentations and supervisees' reactions that might be crucial points of opening to the unconscious, including "innocent" references to the patient's external reality, that otherwise might not be explored.

In all cases there are preferred, repetitive patterns of defense and impulse typical for each patient that emerge, again and again, and require working through. The advantage of dealing with such patterns is that they permit, in the supervisory process, to elucidate some basic criteria for approaching the problem of repetition compulsion, such as, for example, always being alert to what is presently affectively dominant in contrast to assuming that it will be the same content repeated session after session, and what function this repetition may have for the patient–therapist relationship, or in the way in which the patient is dealing with his external reality as an indirect expression of issues in the transference. So that basic learning may evolve in the shifting meanings and functions of repetition compulsion, and this permits the supervisor to evaluate the extent to which the therapist is learning in the process of working through a particular difficulty in his patient's treatment. Throughout time, the supervisor has to assess what learning occurs in the supervisee's understanding of basic principles, and how to apply them in new ways, in contrast to a surface imitation of the supervisor or a rebellious rejection, for whatever reason, of whatever is suggested in the supervisory process. Learning from experience means the supervisee is learning from the interactive relation with the supervisor.

Frequent Problems

Supervision of psychoanalytic candidates within the same psychoanalytic institute represents an optimal situation for the assumption of some basic common approaches to psychoanalytic theory and technique, including the diagnostic evaluation of the patient, the setting up of the psychoanalytic situation, the management of practical administrative details, and dealing with the process of recording and communicating the material of the sessions on the part of the supervisee. Things become less certain when there is a difference between the institutional setting and/or the theoretical orientation of the two parties. What follows is a reflection about frequent problems relating to different backgrounds within the supervisor/supervisee relationship.

As noted above, there are widely divergent assumptions regarding the advantage of a full diagnostic evaluation, indications and contraindications for treatment, prognostic implications, particular conditions under which the treatment can be carried out, and the correspondent careful and detailed diagnostic study and assessment of the patient. In this regard, on one extreme—to which I confess I belong—are therapists and supervisors who would want to have a very clear knowledge of such a diagnostic assessment, including symptomatology, personality structure, history, present life circumstances, and expectations from treatment; on the other extreme, the assumption is that unconscious conflicts are always present and will manifest themselves in their defensive and impulsive nature in any concrete psychoanalytic encounter without undue influence of therapist bias based on the patient's history and real life experiences. This is thought to be "pure psychoanalysis." In any case, I think here supervisor and supervisee have to reach an agreement about what information the supervisor considers essential for his or her initial orientation to their task or the likeliness that such knowledge might be more helpful later on.

A frequent source of confusion is a misunderstanding of the broadly accepted recommendation by Bion (1967) to approach the patient's material "without memory or desire," which is a wonderful definition of an openness to what may emerge in each session but cannot be applied to erase the emergence of both previous knowledge about the patient and of dominant countertransference attitudes in the therapist in the course of the session, part of the total transference/countertransference activation. In other words, a "forced ignorance" in terms of awareness of continuities regarding the developments in a particular patient's treatment throughout time is *not* an indicator of a good psychoanalytic or psychotherapeutic approach.

The agreement between supervisee and supervisor regarding the general information about the patient that is required at the start of the supervision may occasionally become a problem, but, if so, this may be an indication of a specific aspect of the transference developments in the relationship between supervisee and supervisor. This is an important element of the supervisory process that will become particularly relevant at points of the development of "parallel process" (Baudry 1993), that is, the unconscious replication in the relationship between supervisee and supervisor of an unrecognized, and parallel, problem in the transference/countertransference activation with the patient, which reflects specific difficulties in assessing or dealing with the patient's transference. Unconsciously, the supervisee replicates, in his relationship with the supervisor, with reversed roles, the developments in the transference/countertransference with the patient. This may be a problem as well as an important specific contribution of the supervisory process to the learning and potential growth of the therapist, if understood and analyzed.

A general problem for beginning therapists but, in fact, for therapists at all levels of development and in all types of psychoanalytic treatment as well, is the early detection of dominant transferences and their interpretive management. The diagnosis of the transference usually is not too difficult for the supervisee, but when and how to interpret it may become a significant contribution of the supervisory process.

It is very helpful to help the supervisee develop a general mental frame about what an "optimal relationship" between patient and therapist would look like. Ideally, we would assume a patient who trusts the therapist to be open minded, sympathetic, knowledgeable, but not omniscient or omnipotent, with good will and the capacity to help the patient. The patient, in this benevolent and receptive situation, would attempt, in turn, to look into himself, observe what is coming to mind, and attempt to communicate it without being excessively self-condemnatory, trusting in the help he may receive from the therapist. The therapist, of course, should indeed have an interested, open minded, empathic attitude, with a wish to help the patient understand himself.

Against this ideal picture of mutual trust and respect, the reality of the actual limitations in the patient's experience of the therapist and the related interaction becomes the focus of the therapist's attention. It is this discrepancy with the optimal situation and the actual interaction that marks the emergence of the transference and leads to the understanding of what kind of present relationship is now supplanting the ideal one. This basic understanding of how to diagnose transference emergence may or may not be available to the therapist and represents an important task for the supervisor to assess and to consolidate this awareness in the therapist. It is the springboard from which to diagnose and work interpretively with transference activation. How to manage the transference and, particularly, how to interpret it is the most frequent problem in the supervisory process.

The therapist's openness to, and tolerance of, his countertransference reactions is another common problem in the supervisory process (Arlow 1963). As mentioned before, the supervisee must feel a degree of trust and openness to discuss this with the supervisor, and this should not be taken for granted. Sometimes this openness may have to be tactfully established by the supervisor's sensitivity and tactful perception of limits in the supervisee's trust in him. The supervisee's fear of the supervisor's judgment, the necessity of the critical evaluation of the therapist's work, the therapist's wish to fulfill the supervisor's expectations—and, underneath, potentially rebellious attitudes in relation with the supervisor—may reflect transference dispositions of the therapist that affect the supervisory situation. It is the task of the supervisor to attempt to reduce this fear and distrust and to help the supervisee understand that openness to expression of his or her feelings is not only tolerated but encouraged and might be important in the understanding of the transference/countertransference developments in the treatment of the patient.

Usually, angry, aggressive feelings of the therapist towards the patient are not too difficult to ventilate; aggression is easier to ventilate than frank devaluation; however, a disappointed withdrawal from the patient, the therapist's boredom and sense of uselessness, and unimportance of the patient's communication or of therapeutic process itself: this is more difficult to ventilate than straight aggression. And most difficult of all, intense erotic reactions to the patient in the therapist's countertransference may be most difficult to ventilate in the supervisory situation. This requires tact and understanding on the part of the supervisor.

Here, a delicate balance needs to be established between a full exploration of the supervisee's fantasies and feelings towards the patient as it can be used productively to understand the patient's transference, and the supervisor's discretion to refrain from analyzing the therapist's unconscious problems and motivations to avoid transforming the supervisory relationship into a therapeutic one. The supervisor may have to establish subtle limits and suggest that the therapist address these issues in his own therapy—or recommend therapy to address what has emerged as obstacles to therapeutic competence. The interpretation of the patient's negative transference may be particularly difficult for supervisees who experience the patient's attack as directed against them personally and not as transference phenomena, something easy to recognize in theory but difficult to differentiate when confronted with the intensity of negative transference developments. In contrast, the therapist's emphasis on the patient's fear of fully ventilating his hatred in the transference may help the therapist to overcome his own fear of being the recipient of it and to experience tolerating such an attack. This helps the therapist to be able to withstand the temptation to counterattack, to withdraw from the battleground, or to sink into a guilt-laden depression. This entire process is an important aspect of the learning experience in supervision, and the implicit confidence in and support of the therapist's capacity to tolerate and ventilate aggression in patients and self may be an important emotional learning that helps the supervisee to mature and become realistically self-confident.

The supervisory process provides the supervisee the experience to learn the different ways in which unconscious conflicts can be expressed under different structural conditions of the patient's pathology. In the psychoanalysis of a patient with neurotic personality organization, carried out by a candidate in psychoanalytic training, the main channel of communication of the patient's internal world rests with free association. Careful attention to the content of the patient's verbal communication and the nonverbal communication that accompanies it, together with countertransference developments, provides the entrance to the impulse-defense configuration of the predominant conflict. Assuming that the patient is functioning in a relatively stable set of work and personal relationships within a predictable overall environment, absent serious acting out, the analysis of defensive and impulsive processes displayed through free association is dominant and rewards focused attention on it. In patients presenting borderline personality organization with serious disorganization in their environmental functioning (in work or profession, love and sex, social relations and family entanglement), the affectively dominant communication may reside in the combination of intense, rapidly shifting transference developments and acknowledged or split off chaos in the relations between the patient and his psychosocial environment. The analyst's attention, therefore, may have to encompass transference acting out, the combined dynamics of behavioral communication and free association, and the open or hidden processes occurring in the patient's interactions with his environment.

The unconscious past may be replicated dramatically in chaotic and split off expressions in patients' transferential and environmental interactions and, by means of projective identification, omnipotent control, and splitting, may engender a temporary cognitive disorganization or overwhelming emotional experiences in the therapist. Under these circumstances, the supervisory situation may acquire a function of containment that, in fact, implies an intensification of transference and countertransference developments within the supervisory experience itself, an emergent task for the supervisor. Sometimes "parallel process," expressed in an unconscious acting out of transference and countertransference with role reversals in the supervisory situation, dominates the scene and needs to be tactfully explored. Here, the therapist replicates unconsciously the patient's transference in the supervisory relationship while the supervisor identifies with aspects of the therapist's countertransference. When appropriately diagnosed and ventilated by the supervisor, it may become a very helpful learning experience.

A particular problem may occur when there are widely divergent psychotherapeutic approaches between supervisor and supervisee. The supervisor's understanding and empathy with the experiences of the supervisee, together with the tactful clarification and presentation of the different approach the supervisor is presenting, may require time and patience. For example, a psychodynamic psychotherapist starting standard psychoanalytic training may present as an issue the extent to which the therapist should ask direct questions when something the patient is communicating is not clear. It may require an adjustment in the supervisee's thinking to adopt the therapeutic focus on interpreting what prevents the patient from providing clear information, rather than asking direct questions to overcome the problem. Traditional analysis would say that the interpretation of the reason for the patient's shielding some material needs to be explored. But it may be argued that sometimes a direct question permits clarification of an important fact that otherwise may take a month to elucidate, with the possibility of severe acting out hidden behind that lack of clarity. For example, in the analysis of a patient who suddenly changed her job, after 11 years of apparent satisfactory performance, with a statement that she felt "exhausted." Such a vague statement could be taken at face value with the hope that clarity would gradually emerge over time. On the other hand, a direct question as to what was so "exhausting," and why was it so exhausting at this point, might have raised the true cause of what seemed a precipitous decision, namely, the patient's paranoid fears that people were secretly talking about her and criticizing her, a reflection of the developments in the transference at that point of the treatment.

It is true that direct questions may inappropriately guide the patient in a certain direction. For example, the really irrelevant if, unfortunately, frequently asked question "what were you feeling?" or the guiding question "did it not occur to you that…," implying a certain direction in which the therapist is trying to orient the patient, would reflect abandonment of technical neutrality. So, direct questions at times may be very helpful and at other times problematic, and indirectly this entire issue is a reflection on the position of technical neutrality. In the supervisory process, helping the supervisee to achieve and maintain a position of technical neutrality—without its caricature as distance and ambiguity—may be an important learning objective, but it also applies to the supervisor's combining his interest in teaching something new with the respect for where the supervisee comes from.

Technical neutrality, of course, doesn't imply that the therapist have no strong feelings and remain "without memory nor desire" but that the interpretive intervention be carried out from a viewpoint of concerned objectivity. It is not what the therapist experiences but the extent to which he is able to intervene from the position of a "third excluded" observer of the transference/countertransference developments that matters.

This leads to another frequent problem, the difficulty, in the case of psychoanalytic psychotherapy of patients with severe personality disorders, for supervisors to retrain traditional psychodynamic and psychoanalytic candidates to become aware of the importance of the denial of reality (Kernberg 2018). Particularly, candidates in psychoanalytic training may experience pointing to patients' gross denial of reality as contrary to technically neutral interventions, rather than interpreting the mechanism of denial as a fundamental primitive defensive operation related to splitting.

Supervisees usually have little difficulty in learning that an interpretation, in the case of patients with a neurotic personality organization, implies a complex sequence. This sequence starts with their sharing with a patient an observation of a conscious experience or behavior on the patient's part that, however, gives an indication of being a defense against the threat of an opposite, avoided—repressed—one that shows in other aspects of the patient's experience and, particularly, in nonverbal behavior. Clarification of the patient's conscious experience, confrontation with other aspects of this experience that reflect a motivation to protect the patient against an opposite, unknown aspect of his unconscious experience or wishes, constitute the typical sequence of interpretive interventions with patients presenting a neurotic personality organization and predominately high-level repressive mechanisms of defense. The experience with borderline patients, in contrast, permits the supervisee to learn the interpretive process under conditions when what is defended against is conscious, an experience that is affectively disconnected from the opposite predominant experience at that moment in the patient's mind. So that, in this latter case, interpretation implies the connection between conscious but mutually dissociated experiences and the clarification of the motivation for that affective dissociation or mutual denial. This is usually not a difficult learning process.

The problem emerges in the extent to which the therapist may be able to recognize and reveal his countertransference reactions in the course of the analysis of defense and content in the interpretive process. Here, a significant split between what may be called a classic approach and the relationist approach in psychoanalysis characterizes this dilemma: should countertransference be communicated to the patient at certain points or not? In its favor is the possibility of the patient's learning about the effect of his behavior on the therapist and, by implication, the effect of his behavior on other people under related circumstances. In addition, the communication of the countertransference reveals the therapist as a human being and may facilitate a healthy aspect of the patient's identification with the therapist as part of the psychotherapeutic process. The relationship itself becomes a therapeutic factor. Against this viewpoint, however, it may be argued that communication of the countertransference usually precludes the deepening of transference developments, particularly regarding very primitive aspects of aggressive and sexual transference developments, and tends to maintain a "realistic," positive interpersonal relationship that interferes with full deployment of the analysis of transference in depth. In addition, in the case of severe psychopathology, where the importance of the patient's learning about the effects of his behavior is maximal, the successive alternative, reciprocal projection of self and object representations in the case of each activated conflict facilitates the patient's identification with the experience that, at other times, the therapist may experience in the countertransference, thus facilitating a learning process without the therapist having to communicate his countertransference experience. In agreement with this latter position, I believe that countertransference should not be communicated, and this is part of my own supervisory attitude. However, I believe the therapist should learn that there are times when it may be perfectly appropriate to communicate to the patient the therapist's emotional experience, if that experience is a natural expression of what the patient himself has been implying, thus heightening the understanding of what is going on in the patient's mind.

For example, a patient mentioned, in the course of a session, that she was annoyed with her boyfriend because he had shared a photograph of her posing naked that she had given to him with a friend of his. The patient had learned this from the girlfriend of that friend. She mentioned it with a slight sign of irritation and went on to discuss other subjects. In supervision, the therapist mentioned to me that he was quite shocked at the boyfriend's behavior, which seemed radically different from how the patient had described their love relation before, and he was troubled by his patient's subdued reaction to this infringement of their intimacy. But he felt he should not share his countertransference with the patient. I suggested that it might have been helpful to express his surprise at his patient's lack of reaction to this very inappropriate behavior and her lack of reflection about what this behavior revealed about their relationship. This, of course, illustrates both sharing of the therapist's reaction and the beginning interpretation of the patient's denial of reality. Interpretation of the denial of reality often is misunderstood as a cognitive-supportive intervention, but it does not involve an instruction of how the patient should behave, but, rather, it focuses on a motivated ignorance or naiveté, a psychogenic blindness.

I have explored frequent problems in the supervisory process dealing with the essential instruments of psychoanalytic technique, that is, interpretation, transference analysis, technical neutrality, and countertransference developments, in addition to the importance of the relatively neglected aspect of the denial of reality in cases of severe psychopathology. Now I would like to point to more general issues in the supervisory process regarding the objectives of the treatment, the realistic expectations of patient and therapist, and the implicit expectations of what may be called a "good life" for the patient that frames concrete therapeutic goals. I am referring here to the frequent self-restriction of patients' expectations for themselves and from life that becomes a major issue in masochistic and generally self-destructive psychopathology but may reflect a much more general problem in terms of the unavoidable conflicts between love and aggression, particularly self-directed aggression as a universal challenge. This problem may emerge even with better functioning patients, who may reveal limitations in what they expect as a satisfactory work situation, and in their efforts to obtain optimal educational and social support to be able to achieve a broad spectrum of possibilities in work or profession. It also refers to the resignation to a less than fully satisfactory experience in a love relationship, in the expectations from a marriage, and the search for general gratification in "non-survival" activity, from hobbies to engagement in culture, knowledge, sport, and other areas of interest. In short, what are the patient's aspirations and possibilities, in work and profession, love and sex, social life and creativity?

Therapists should resolve in their own mind what are the limits they see in their patients' improvement as part of the treatment, what is the best that the patient may reasonably expect for his life? The supervisor, I believe, should attempt to invite the therapist to put himself/herself "into the body" of their patient, imagining, for example, that the therapist would wake up one morning finding himself in the body of the patient, in the exact life situation in which the patient is involved. Putting oneself in the patient's shoes and asking, "what should I now do within this new situation in which I am to make my life as good as it can be?"

This may be an important exercise, particularly with severely self-destructive or self-limiting patients who unconsciously attempt to convince the therapist that they cannot go beyond the point in which they are, that they are hopeless, that they can expect nothing from life. This exercise may help the therapist to pinpoint the areas of self-restrictions, the rationalization of self-defeating behavior; the patient's resignation to situations that objectively don't conform to their potential. Carrying out such a process at the beginning of the treatment may help to clarify the relation between optimal treatment goals and the realistic goals that the patient has traced for himself and that the therapist has traced before this particular exercise.

Such an imaginary travel into the existential reality of his patient may permit the therapist to question the patient's acceptance of his/her present situation in love or marriage, at work or profession, the attitude of the patient toward his own area of creative activity, the patient's relationship to friendships and changing life challenges.

This exercise allows the therapist to realistically evaluate the extent to which there are unconscious, conflictual motivational issues that prevent the patient from moving into the desired direction, and it may free the therapist from being contaminated by the patient's self-restrictive constraints. Suggesting such an exercise challenges the therapist to explore potential limitations in his/her own view of what may be expected realistically in life, what can be expected in a good love relation, how does one assess whether one is stuck in a bad work situation, and when it is worthwhile to be contented with the present or be adventurous in looking for alternative possibilities. It may lead to an open discussion of life goals and philosophical approaches to life on the part of the supervisor and the supervisee and raises again the issue of the extent to which the supervisee has to be helped to find his own ways in contrast to the supervisor's imposing his way, and the extent of change the therapist attempts to achieve with his patient. This is one more reason to carefully explore the reality of the social environment in which the patient develops his potential, as well as facing his limitations (Kernberg 2018).

And the therapist's own self-imposed limitations, restrictions in his love life or professional arrangements, may emerge as part of the management of potential limits and openings in the life of his patient. Under optimal circumstances, the supervisory experience, over an extended period of time, may lead to these existential questions involving dimensions of the therapist's countertransference that transcend particular treatment situations and also, at times, for the supervisor as well. Every supervisory process exploring the consequences of the treatment for the life of the patient necessarily touches universal human aspirations, possibilities, and limitations and opens opportunities for growth of therapist and supervisor.

In an optimal, long-term supervision the supervisor may have the opportunity to help the therapist explore his own vision about normality and pathology, life goals and their limitations, the understanding and tolerance for alternative lifestyles. The mutual confidence and trust between therapist and supervisor is essential to fully explore transference and countertransference related to a case but, at its best, also extends into existential and philosophical aspects of the relationship with all our patients.

Limitations

Perhaps the most painful limitation of the supervisory experience arises with supervisees who lack the capacity to enter empathically into the life of their patients: supervisees whose intelligence or personality pathology presents limits that cannot be effectively dealt with in the supervisory process. Usually professional training guarantees a sufficient intellectual capacity for carrying out psychotherapeutic work on the part of those who are interested in that subject. Unfortunately, however, because of the combination of unfortunate circumstances of undiagnosed limitations of intellectual capability and motivational misperceptions of the nature of this work, the actual field of psychodynamic psychotherapy turns out to be beyond some trainees' capacity. One has to differentiate these cases from severe narcissistic pathology, where often very high intellectual capacities and intense motivational commitment enter into severe contradiction to the lack of capacity for empathy related to the narcissistic deterioration of the supervisee's world of internal object relations. Sometimes, regrettably, the psychotherapeutic profession is narcissistically perceived as a road to an elitist grandiosity and superiority. In the case of intellectual limitations, or those limitations derived from characterological pathology, helping therapists to work with patients in other professional areas may provide a satisfactory alternative, at least as a recommendation when things don't go well.

In the case of severe narcissistic pathology, the optimal recommendation is a personal psychoanalysis or psychoanalytic psychotherapy, and this may also be the recommendation for trainees with obsessive-compulsive personality structures highly motivated to become psychoanalytic psychotherapists. At the same time, it needs to be said that, sometimes, psychotherapists with borderline personality organization and various types of personality syndromes may become excellent psychotherapists as long as they are free from antisocial features and have a capacity and commitment to consistent and systematic work.

Does psychoanalysis help to become a good psychotherapist? Is it indispensable for becoming a good psychoanalyst or psychoanalytic psychotherapist? Is it possible to become a good psychoanalytic psychotherapist without personal analysis or therapy? These questions are consistently raised, and, as long as we don't have good empirical evidence to answer them, we can only provide our clinical experience. In my own experience, a personal psychoanalysis or long-term, intensive psychoanalytic psychotherapy is extremely helpful, and, for most, indispensable to becoming a good psychotherapist. However, there are some very good psychoanalytic psychotherapists I have had the opportunity to supervise and to work with in professional settings who have had no personal therapeutic experience at all! There are some frighteningly normal people who are able to do it without having been in treatment themselves, obviously persons with great emotional maturity and an unusual capacity for empathy. In most cases, I believe, psychoanalytic psychotherapy or a personal analysis is of great help, and in the case of narcissistic psychopathology an absolutely essential precondition for being able to work well in this field.

Can psychoanalysis limit one's potential for psychotherapeutic work outside psychoanalysis proper? I believe that the old assumption that a trained psychoanalyst can do any kind of psychoanalytic psychotherapy as well is disappearing. New, specialized models of psychoanalytic psychotherapy, such as transference-focused psychotherapy, clearly require specialized training, and psychoanalytic institutes should provide them. Unfortunately, there are some psychoanalysts whose personal rigidity makes it difficult for them to learn and employ the specific technical approaches of modified psychoanalytic psychotherapies such as transference-focused psychotherapy. A large majority of psychoanalytically trained therapists, however, are able to learn various modalities of psychoanalytic psychotherapy in addition to standard psychoanalysis within their particular orientation. I have found that psychoanalysts trained within the Kleinian tradition are particularly able to employ systematic transference and countertransference analysis under a variety of therapeutic circumstances and with severely regressed patients.

Perhaps the most important unresolved issue affecting supervision is the serious contradiction between the fundamental importance of the su-

pervisory experience in the training of psychoanalysts and psychoanalytic psychotherapists, on the one hand, and the unresolvable problem of
those trainees who simply are not able to acquire the corresponding
skills and who, for various characterological reasons, simply are unable
to overcome a very definite limit to their capacity to respond appropriately to what they may diagnose correctly as their difficulties but without
being able to influence them. Such difficulties are evinced by candidates
who get paralyzed by certain forms of sadistic transferences, who find
deep levels of sadomasochistic sexuality in patients' communications
difficult or impossible to understand or to handle. Sometimes, candidates with powerful obsessive defenses against intense affect activation
present significant limitations in their empathic responses.

Supervisors may recommend that, after supervision reaches a stand-
still, the candidate shift to be supervised by somebody else, and the
same paralyzing process may repeat itself. Institutionally fostered silence regarding a trainee's incompetence may be secretly recognized by
the supervisory community but encounters institutional lack of courage
to confront the candidate. The slow process in candidates' advancing
throughout the various stages of psychoanalytic institutions' training
may extend this frustrating, failing supervisory situation over several
years, and faculty's guilt feelings regarding candidates who were not
able to "make it" interferes with a direct ventilation of the problem. This
leads to "compassionate graduation," an institutional willingness to
bury the whole problem, with the uneasy sense that quality control has
not been maintained. Eventually, in order to be able to solve this on an
institutional basis, a total review of the educational process is needed.
For the individual supervisor faced with the ethical problem of helping
a candidate to honestly face a problem, this is a difficult responsibility.

Paradoxically, because of its public nature, group supervision may be
the most powerful contribution to highlighting what is essential in the
supervisory process, as well as exposing limits to the learning process in
individual members of the group. I am not referring to critically exposing individual supervisees in terms of their problems in the supervisory
process but the implicit highlighting of these difficulties as the entire
group advances in the understanding of an unconscious conflict represented in the patient material examined by the group. As mentioned before, the different responses, within the group of supervisees, to the
material presented by one of them, usually tends to highlight the complexity of transference and countertransference in the patient's material, and the clarification of the criteria by which what is essential and
what needs to be focused upon emerge clearly in the work of the group.
In the process, basic principles of technique and priorities in the analytic
management of the material will become a shared learning process. For
this purpose, however, it is important that the supervisor—the leader of
the supervisory group—apply group techniques, stimulating the partic-

ipation of individual members as well as being able to analyze the development of basic themes within the group process that emerge in the supervision of an individual case.

Seminars on psychoanalytic and psychotherapeutic technique need to be supported by a significant number of group supervisors. I believe this aspect of the training program has not been sufficiently prioritized in the training program of many psychoanalytic institutions.

Returning once more to the essential task of supervision of psychoanalytic treatment: the objective is to help the supervisee develop his or her own integrated frame of reference that permits to organize the many simultaneous impressions, the many different emotional experiences and facts that emerge in every session of psychotherapy. To be able to respond in a focused way that does justice to the intuitive organizing of all these experiences in the supervisee's mind requires the gradual maturing of an integrated concept of technique. To achieve such an integrative process throughout time, the supervisor has to clarify his own internal technical frame, and this growth process within the supervisor is perhaps the most exciting consequence of carrying out a supervisory function, together with the gratification of the learning process and the growth of the supervisee. At best, supervision may become a dialogue about life.

References

Arlow JA: The supervisory situation. J Am Psychoanal Assoc 11:576–594, 1963

Baudry FD: The personal dimension and management of the supervisory situation with a special note on the parallel process. Psychoanal Q 62:588–614, 1993

Bion WR: Notes on memory and desire. Psychoanalytic Forum 2:272–273, 279–290, 1967

Blomfield O: Psychoanalytic supervision: an overview. Int Rev Psychoanal 12:401–409, 1985

Greenberg L: On transference and countertransference and the technique of supervision, in Supervision and Its Vicissitudes. Edited by Martindale B, Möner M, Rodriguez MEC, et al. London, Karnac, 1997, pp 1–24

Kernberg OF: Psychoanalytic supervision: the supervisor's tasks. Psychoanal Q 79:603–627, 2010

Kernberg OF: The denial of reality, in Treatment of Severe Personality Disorders: Resolution of Aggression and Recovery of Eroticism. Washington, DC, American Psychiatric Association Publishing, 2018, pp 251–263

Tuckett D: Does anything go? Toward a framework for the more transparent assessment of psychoanalytic competence. Int J Psychoanal 86:31–49, 2005

Yerushalmi H: On the presence and absence of supervisors. Am J Psychoanal 79(3):398–415, 2019

PART III

Specific Psychopathologies

CHAPTER 7

Psychodynamics and Treatment of Schizoid Personality Disorders

The study of the schizoid personality disorder is complicated by the discrepancy between the precise definition of the descriptive characteristics of the schizoid personality in classical descriptive psychiatry—that is, the observable behavior defining the syndrome without a major exploration of the underlying dynamics—and the psychoanalytic exploration of schizoid mechanisms of defense and their clinical development. Psychoanalytic explorations have provided in-depth analysis of schizoid defenses, their underlying psychodynamics, and their corresponding intrapsychic conflicts but in the context of a rather diffuse, poorly circumscribed definition of this syndrome. Schizoid defensive organization and the syndrome described in clinical psychiatry no longer coincide. It seems important to first define the descriptive characteristics of the schizoid personality disorder and to then explore the typical corresponding uncon-

Translated from Damman G, Kernberg OF (eds): *Schizoidie und Schizoide Persönlichkeitsstörung*. Stuttgart, Germany, Kohlhammer, 2019, pp 187–201. Used with permission.

scious defensive operations and respective conflicts while differentiating this approach from other ways in which schizoid defensive mechanisms have been explored in the psychoanalytic literature without regard to the corresponding personality structure. Psychoanalytic studies have expanded the concept of schizoid defense but have lost, in the process, the precise correspondence between unconscious defensive dynamics and descriptive psychopathology.

Perhaps the essential manifestation of this discrepancy is the descriptive characteristic of the schizoid personality described in DSM-5 (American Psychiatric Association 2013, p. 653): These patients "appear to lack a desire for intimacy, seem indifferent to opportunities to develop close relationships," while, from a psychodynamic perspective, schizoid patients are described as frequently evincing a dynamic of desperate desire and search for intimacy and closeness and a simultaneous fear of being overwhelmed and overtaken by another person, a constellation that has been most clearly examined by Fairbairn (1954), Guntrip (1969), and McWilliams (2011). The psychoanalytic development of contemporary object relations theory pertaining to the defensive mechanisms and split object relations of the early "paranoid-schizoid position" (Klein 1946) used and expanded Fairbairn's concepts in describing a more general early psychological constellation common to human development in general and pathologically exacerbated in a broad spectrum of psychopathology. This broader consideration of paranoid and schizoid mechanisms has diluted the relationship between the specific schizoid mechanisms of schizoid personality and the general schizoid mechanisms that are part of the paranoid-schizoid position. What must be clarified is a more specific view of the dynamics of the schizoid personality disorder and its specific defensive operations. Practically, the splitting operations that separate idealized and persecutory internalized object relations typical of the earliest levels of development need to be differentiated from the generalized fragmentation of affective experience, typical for the schizoid personality disorder, that constitutes both an extreme form of splitting and a clearly specific defensive operation that Melanie Klein simply considered as corresponding to a form of extreme anxiety.

Briefly, the descriptive characteristics of schizoid personality disorder (Akhtar 1992; McWilliams 2011) include social withdrawal; a tendency to social isolation; lack of intimate relationships; hypersensitivity to the interactions with others, with an exaggerated sensitivity to aversive, hostile implications in such interactions; and a vulnerability to feeling misunderstood, rejected, or hurt. The latter influences the social withdrawal of these patients and complicates their heightened awareness of the expression of others' feelings, the meaning of subtle aspects of the behavior of others, and their interactions with them. These patients attempt to retreat into internal self-affirmation as protection against social rejection and mistreatment. This fosters development of an internal fantasy world that replicates their real and desired experiences, while their objective interactional life appears impoverished.

The psychodynamic exploration of their fantasy life reveals desperate desires to engage in close and dependent relationships and, at the same time, the fear that in such relationships they would be subjected to an overwhelming effort of control and determination by others. In contrast to empathic and tender relationships in reality, these patients may present dissociated sexual and aggressive relations that appear to have an impulsive as well as a dissociated character and seem widely disconnected from their conscious experiences and fantasy life. They show a lack of modulated affect activation, with a general fragmentation or dispersal of both positive and negative affects, so that not only others but they themselves experience confusion regarding their own momentary affect state or mood. This alternates with the sudden explosion of powerful dissociative positive and negative affects, which may be reflected in impulsive behaviors that seem in strong contrast to the patients' habitual demeanor.

From a psychodynamic perspective, the predominant conflicts these patients evince with their internal object representations and their parental objects in reality are characterized by the fact that they cannot tolerate the corresponding intensive affective dispositions. When intense affective experiences emerge, there follows an immediate process of a typical dispersal or dilution of affect that results in a profound fragmentation of all psychic experiences, affects, and thought processes, as well as the affect proper, and leads to cognitive and emotional confusion. Patients are not clear about what they are experiencing and center themselves in a situation of internal void and lack of any internal guidance about what their affective relation is to the significant other with whom they may be involved at that moment. In short, whatever specific oedipal or preoedipal unconscious conflicts are activated in patients, the structural disposition of schizoid personality disorder expresses a defensive reaction against the full affective experience of the corresponding conflict by means of a methodical fragmentation of cognitive and affective experience on the one hand and development of a particular state of total isolation from internal relations with significant others on the other. This emotional situation then leads to an intense desire for contact, dependency, and a loving relationship while, simultaneously, the fear of being overtaken, invaded, and totally controlled by an alien mind paralyzes their search for any real contact with significant others. This specific defensive constellation of schizoid personality disorder needs to be differentiated clearly from the general paranoid-schizoid position described by Melanie Klein, in which full affective experience of a positive libidinal nature is clearly split off from a purely negative, hostile set of affective experiences and internalized object relations, together with the corresponding mechanisms of primitive idealization, projective identification, denial, devaluation, omnipotence, and omnipotent control.

The following clinical cases illustrate this specific relationship between descriptive psychopathology of schizoid personality disorder and the defensive operations involved in the typical management of the corresponding, dominant unconscious conflicts.

THE CASE OF JENNIFER

The descriptive diagnosis was a schizoid personality disorder. This was a woman in her early twenties who had always been shy and somewhat withdrawn. This became more accentuated during high school years and led to her increasing social isolation in the last 2 years of high school and the first 2 years of college. At the end of that second year, she became unable to continue her studies because of an increasing social withdrawal and difficulty in maintaining an appropriate intensity of studies and preparation for exams. Over the next year, she increased her practice of discreet self-mutilating behavior in the form of minor, superficial cuts all over her body. She became fascinated with watching drops of blood emerging in those cuts of the skin and claimed that it reduced her almost-constant sense of anxiety. She had been able to date briefly during the last year of high school, but these relationships did not last long because of her apparent total lack of interest in any sexual intimacy. She tolerated some degree of petting without any apparent emotional participation or sexual excitement, which contributed to the failure of her relations with the young men.

The dominant family dynamics included a powerful, controlling, yet seductive father who seemed warmly interested in her and yet overwhelmingly domineering. He attempted to prescribe her behavior in all details and discuss what he thought her future professional orientation should be. The mother, complementing this behavior of the father, supported his overall control but maintained a cold distance to her daughter that was complicated by the mother's attempts to influence the patient by systematically raising guilt feelings whenever she seemed opposed to family customs, rules, and regulations. A brief period of rebelliousness in early adolescence had been followed by a quiet submission at home while Jennifer's isolation at school increased, and the self-cutting behavior emerged during the later high school years. Her childhood history revealed a period in which the patient had become very close to her father, much closer than had been the case for her older brother and sister, but then she developed serious conflicts regarding his efforts to control her and her mother's support of that behavior that led her to withdraw from both of them.

I treated this patient with transference-focused psychotherapy (TFP) (Yeomans et al. 2015) in two weekly sessions while arranging for her to gradually take some college courses, with a plan to expand to full resumption of her college education in later stages of the treatment. During the early months of the treatment, the patient talked with an expression of disgust about her father's particular behavior, his attempts to show emotional interest by touching her hand, which she found disgusting. She complained about his embracing her against her wishes. At the same time, she evinced a resentful rejection of her mother. She felt she hated her mother but also felt guilty about the intensity of her hatred. As the treatment progressed over the first 6 months, her communications gradually decreased, longer silences developed, and her language seemed increasingly fragmented. I had a growing sense that her demeanor reflected a growing distance and indifference, that she was just going through the motions of free association in the sessions, that had an effect of distancing me as well from the relationship with her. I became distracted and repeatedly experienced brief fantasies that seemed not to have anything to do with the patient nor with this immediate situation. There were sessions in which I experienced a vague, subtle erotic quality in her behavior and her interaction with me, but this quality would disperse as soon as it appeared in the session.

It was in this context that, on one occasion, I had the sudden, intense memory of a film I had seen many months earlier, *Investigation of a Citizen Without Suspicion*, in which a district attorney, charged with identifying a murderer who killed his female victims while having sexual relations with them, was revealed to be the murderer himself. I remembered one scene in which a woman was sitting on him sexually and, as she reached orgasm, he pulled a knife and cut her throat, causing blood to run over her breasts. This image emerged strongly in my mind with a combination of excitement and disgust. The strangeness and intensity of this memory became an alarm signal regarding what was going on in the transference and countertransference. Now I became alert to the combination of occasional subtle erotic manifestations in the sessions; the patient's self-cutting activity, which had increased again; and her description of the disgusting "sexual" approach from her father. I raised the question, over the next few weeks, as to what extent her profound distance in the hours protected her from frightening fantasies about me.

The patient finally was able to tell me that she had powerful fantasies involving a wish that I would shoot her. The idea was that, if I were to kill her, I would become a murderer and would have to think of her for the rest of my life, and then she would be united with me forever! That fantasy gave her an enormous satisfaction and was expressed with such an intensity and conviction that this was a reasonable way to obtain a permanent, close relationship with me that it was difficult, at first, for me to explore the terribly self-destructive nature of that fantasy. It opened up the exploration of the patient's powerful masochistic relationship with an aggressive and seductive father image and reflected a deep sense of guilt and fear over the internal persecution by a revengeful mother. She revealed, in short, an aggressive primitive oedipal constellation that proved to be the dominant unconscious conflict with which she was struggling.

I have to stress that the first few months of this treatment were characterized by sessions in which her free association seemed to reveal total dispersal of cognitive thinking, isolated pieces of memory, fantasy, or observations that only contributed to a chaotic impossibility to diagnose a

dominant subject. All of this was augmented by an ambiance of the patient's emotional distance and unavailability. During those early months,
any effort to clarify what she was talking about or to assert my presence
by expressing the intensity of my wish to understand what was happening would lead her immediately to withdraw. It almost felt as if she was
"training" me to maintain distance to avoid further, more extreme withdrawal on her part. A massive schizoid defense operated during these
first 6 months of treatment, and the main conflict with which she was
struggling became only gradually apparent through the rather extreme
countertransference development I described. Opening up the regressive oedipal conflict in the transference transitorily resolved this severe
fragmentation of cognitive processes and emotional distance. Later on,
these defensive operations reappeared again and again over a period of
several years as we advanced our understanding of other specific aspects
of her infantile conflicts and their impact on her present life.

THE CASE OF SARAH

Sarah was a woman in her early thirties. She had graduated from a distinguished college where she had specialized in the literature of a particular non-Western culture. She had graduated with significant approval
of her work by a leading specialist in that field but then failed to take up
any position that would have permitted her to continue either teaching
or do scholarly work in her field. She had, in contrast, routinely taken up
entry-level secretarial administrative positions in various organizations,
only to leave each one after a few months due to boredom. In this way,
she drifted from job to job, all of which were beneath her capabilities and
educational level. She worked to maintain herself, with additional financial support from her parents, and seemingly without any particular interest or dedication. This was a great disappointment for her father, who
earlier had been supportive of her but who ended up saddened and began to limit their relationship, which she resented bitterly. Her mother
was a socially rather withdrawn person whom the patient described as
viewing her roles as wife and mother of several daughters as an obliga-
tion she was willing to fulfill, showing little interest in the development
of her children once they had left home. Within that rather loveless environment there was a prevalent sense of responsibility and tolerance of
fulfilling all social obligations but in the context of an overall absence of
any deep involvement. That combination of tolerance and indifference
also was communicated in the striking way in which the patient conveyed her family background.

    Sarah came to treatment because of a chronic characterologically
based depression and a history of longstanding unhappy sexual relationships with both men and women. Although she seemed predominantly
interested in heterosexual relationships, she expressed her openness to
relations with both sexes. She had indicated intense dependency needs
from whomever she was involved with but also easy disappointment
that would lead her to withdraw. Thus, she gave the person she was involved with the feeling that she was rejecting him or her and that she

lacked a loving commitment, which led her partners to end the relationship and left her disappointed. She believed that she really never had fallen in love deeply.

My first impression was that she probably presented a narcissistic personality disorder of the relatively less frequent kind, presenting with social withdrawal rather than overtly overestimating her own importance and superiority. That impression, however, was rapidly corrected by her deep suffering from her lack of connection with others, although she was not able, apparently, to show this in any way that would communicate her wishes to others. To the contrary, she conveyed an attitude of critical rejection whenever she felt something was wrong in the way she was being treated. She conveyed what seemed at first a relative sexual freedom and openness in terms of enjoying her sexual relations with both men and women, but these turned out to be erotic experiences that did not lead to more emotional intimacy. She was willing to engage in relationships with a lack of expectation of such emotional intimacy, as though sexual intimacy was the way of demonstrating and maintaining an intimate relationship without any major emotional involvement from either partner, yet she felt terribly alone. Her depression centered around that sense of aloneness, despite the evident opportunities she had for social engagements and relationships, particularly in connection with her intellectual interests. However, she was neglecting her professional involvement with non-Western cultures.

In the transference, what predominated from early on was her sense that the nature of her treatment implied a total lack of my presence. As far as she was concerned, I wasn't there. She was in analysis for four sessions a week. Initially, I had wondered whether a person with such strong schizoid features would tolerate an analytic situation. I had considered that the stability of her character pathology and her relative ego strength were in many ways sufficient for undergoing a standard psychoanalytic experience. On the couch, however, she experienced my lack of ongoing responses to her comments as a terrible withdrawal and implicit rejection, a distancing and indifference on my part that gave her a sense of aloneness and confusion that she could barely tolerate. My efforts to explore what kind of internal relationship I reflected in this experience, with the tentative assumption that early conflicts with a rejecting mother image might be a dominant issue, only led her to develop a frightening sense that I was bombarding her with bookish, intellectual hypotheses that had nothing to do with her.

Whenever I seemed to her to show an intense interest and conveyed a sense of understanding about what was going on in her, she reacted with a panicky sense of being "brainwashed." It took a long period of time for me to become aware, in my growing frustration over her apparent unchanging emotional unavailability in the sessions, that behind her experience of me as either totally indifferent or threateningly invasive was her sense that my indifference merely disguised a profound hatred of her. She believed I defended against this hatred by assuming indifference but could not avoid occasional aggressive invasiveness in the way I treated her. It turned out that her intolerance of her own feelings of ha-

tred toward her cold mother and her weak father, who had not been able
to supply the love she needed, was expressed through a total dispersal
or fragmentation of any affects. Emotional fragmentation, the schizoid
defense against affective experience, interfered with the projective identification of hatred that she projected onto me and implied an omnipotent control of the total therapeutic situation. The patient could tolerate
a wish to depend on a loving object, but the profound conviction that
such an object did not exist, and that her own need for love would be
lost, maintained her own emotional dispersal as well as the incapacity
to recognize anything but invasive hatred in anyone else's approach.
My suggestion of any specific meaning to Sarah's confused emotional
experience appeared to her as an invasive attack.

In this case, profound frustration of the earliest needs for a securely
dependent relationship, and the corresponding activation of revengeful
resentment, was further complicated by Sarah's intolerance of the ordinary paranoid-schizoid defenses. The lack of any compensating good pa-
ternal relationship interfered with establishing split-off idealized and
persecutory internal object relations. This was replaced by the specific
schizoid conviction that no trustworthy object existed and the dismantling fragmentation of any capacity for experiencing intense affective reactions. Gradually, in the treatment, it became possible for Sarah to
tolerate her intense resentment of her mother and the reasons for her immediate withdrawal upon any minor frustration, experienced rejection, or
shortcoming in my responses to her. Gradually, intense demandingness
and angry expectations for my immediate response to her experienced
needs replaced the distance and the fragmentation of the sessions. Her tolerance of intense hostile demandingness and her revengeful, unconscious
destruction of what she received because she felt it was given under force-
ful demand could be painfully worked through in the transference.

THE CASE OF ROBERT

Robert was a 19-year-old adolescent who came to treatment because of
aggressive behavior at home and at school, general social withdrawal
from friends and family, and an attitude of "leave me alone," which had
threatening implications. He was prepared to counterattack anybody
who provoked or challenged him. He had attacked several people verbally and had been physically menacing, including a few relatively mild
physical struggles at school. His attacks on his parents were limited to
verbal explosions. At school, he responded well to some teachers and
had been able to achieve good grades but had failed in other classes and
had expressed provocative behavior toward teachers and other students.
He evinced a general paranoid rigidity in all his interactions and was referred to treatment because of the growing concerns of both the school
and his parents. His behavioral problems were increasing, and his senior high school work was deteriorating.

Robert's father was an extremely dominant, explosive, distrustful
individual who chronically challenged school authorities and his son's
therapists but was basically interested in helping his son normalize his

behavior. I found it possible to work with him and with the mother, who impressed me as depressed and relatively indifferent, having resigned herself to the aggressive behavior of her child. She was submissive to her husband but with an attitude of hoping that, by being so, she would be "left in peace." On mental status examination, the patient appeared paranoid, defiant, and explosive. In the early sessions of therapy he oscillated between what seemed an extreme fearfulness, an attitude as though he were a prisoner being interrogated by police authorities, and a threatening oppositionalism that induced a countertransference fear of assault in me. He was treated with TFP, two sessions per week. He was given the diagnosis of paranoid personality disorder and moderate, characterological-based depression. In the course of the treatment he gradually stabilized in what seemed a marked distancing and emotional emptiness. He conveyed a sense of internal confusion and lack of contact with me that seemed to replicate the withdrawal from social contacts he had experienced over the past 2 years.

In a typical session, he arrived dressed all in black, looking somewhat threatening, and then sat down with an expression of being tired, exhausted, and, finally, fearful and uncertain in his face and gestures. His communications revealed an incapacity to convey any specific emotional relationship with anybody else, except the general experience of not knowing what he was interested in or what he wanted to do. He seemed ready, at any moment, to shift from that exhausted, hopeless position to a defiant withdrawal into a challenging hyperalertness towards me. I clearly sensed that he was struggling against a consistent fearfulness of aggression breaking out in him or in the people surrounding him, without his being able to explain why; the fearfulness about anger could not be traced to any specific experience. He also oscillated between moments when he thought I would attack him and other times when he perceived me as not dangerous at all but, rather, indifferent and uninvolved. I think both of us were colluding in an experience of shared meaningless that would lead to no consequence of any kind.

It was interesting that the analysis of the transferential implications of the feared hateful interaction between him and me, while clearly related to a resentful, fearful, and rebellious attitude toward his explosive and domineering father, also seemed to reveal a specific defensive function against intolerable homosexual wishes toward the father that he could not tolerate. Any effort to clarify this aspect of his difficulties unavoidably ended in a general lack of feeling, a loss of all emotional meaning in our interaction. I then would experience a sense of confusing emptiness, and Robert, in turn, would confront me with an empty smile or, rather, what may be described as a slightly ironic confirmation of his belief that nothing further could be understood or learned from his situation. Eventually, I developed a clearer sense that I was enacting the role of an indifferent mother while the patient was unconvincingly attempting to demonstrate that his indifference and withdrawal were the only rational response to such a frustrating, painful situation.

Thus, the general fragmentation of the patient's affective experience, leading to his evolving sense of emptiness and meaningless in the hours, became the only alternative to an angry, dangerous outburst of rage at his father. His experience of me as equally unavailable and distant, without any hope of improving our relationship, illustrated his regression to a schizoid organization that also corresponded to the serious social withdrawal he had experienced in recent years. Many months of work were necessary before he could tolerate and experience more directly the wish for a loving relationship with his father, while recognizing the impossibility of obtaining that in the past, and the deeper wish for a loving relationship with me as a combined primitive mother-father figure who nonetheless seemed unobtainable because of his deep conviction of my unavailability, my indifferent rejection, and even my disgust toward him as an early mother image.

Psychodynamic Considerations and Treatment

It was Fairbairn (1954) who originally observed the splitting mechanisms involved in the internalization of early idealized and persecutory, good and bad object relations as an essential aspect of the predominance of fragmented emotional experiences in schizoid personalities and the affective impoverishment of a central ego resulting from the split-off and mutually dissociated idealized and persecutory segments of experience. He also concluded that schizoid patients would show the combination of an intense need for the love of an ideal object, a profound conviction of that object's emotional unavailability and of the futility of expecting that object to be responsive to the patient's love, and the related despair and consequential psychological retreat. His analysis of the schizoid mechanism led Melanie Klein (1946, 1952, 1958) to expand the definition of the earliest paranoid position to the paranoid-schizoid position and facilitated the full development of the Kleinian theory of early developmental stages. Guntrip (1961, 1969) expanded the specific findings from Fairbairn in his clinical studies, stressing the early pathology in the relationship to the mother. From a contemporary perspective, the predominance of schizoid defensive mechanisms clearly indicates a lack of resolution of the earliest conflicts of attachment and their consequences for the erotic life of these patients. The development of the knowledge regarding Klein's paranoid-schizoid position gradually expanded the concept of schizoid phenomena to a broad pathology—the fixation at an early stage of mental development with a maintained dissociation between idealized and persecutory mental segments—and led to the relative neglect of analyzing specific features of the schizoid personality in contrast to the general schizoid position of early development. The schizoid personality disorder illustrates how early conflicts regarding frustrated dependency needs, the fear of being invaded or taken over, and the contamination of the oedipal situation by these early conflicts determine the pathological development of these patients and lead to the dominance of a specific defensive schizoid structure.

The three cases I mentioned illustrate the commonality of this basic schizoid structure, which includes a generalized fragmentation of affect, the conviction of the unavailability of the love object, fear over being invaded or taken over, and a refuge into an internal withdrawal and a confusional, fragmented self state that assures protection against any specific affective relationship. Within this basic common defensive structure, however, differentiated transference dispositions emerged in these patients: in the case of Jennifer, the predominance of the severely masochistic orientation in her relation to both parents; in the case of Sarah, the defense against her extreme ambivalence relating to an insecure and severely conflictual dependency; and in the case of Robert, the hateful oedipal competition and his struggle against homosexual submission to an oedipal rival. These three cases thus illustrate different emotional conflicts submerged behind the protective dominance of the schizoid defensive structure, while sharing the presence of severe early pathology of internalized object relations and identity diffusion (Kernberg 2011). Their treatment included, eventually, the need to resolve this identity diffusion by integrating the conflictual, idealized, and persecutory segments of mental experience. The dissolution or dispersal of dominant affective experiences apparently erases any specific object relationship in terms of an affective linkage between self- and object representations, and this constitutes the specific difference of the schizoid structure from all other borderline pathology. The clarification and resolution of this schizoid dispersal in the transference relies strongly on countertransference analysis and the parallel analysis of these patients' external reality and world of fantasies—when it can be recovered.

The question may be raised: What is it that determines the potential for this affective dispersal or dissolution that seems so sharply contrasting with powerful early activation of affect dispositions? Is it a consequence of a particular genetic, constitutionally determined temperamental dysfunction, or of a particular pathology of attachment processes? Clearly this chronic schizoid disposition differs from the temporary depersonalization experiences that are connected with the activation of moods. Moods also may present with a dispersal of affective experience, but without eliminating the specific nature of the affect involved and without the parallel fragmentation of self-experience and thought processes. This dispersal also differs from narcissistic devaluation of object relations because schizoid personality has a highly differentiated capability of intuitively assessing affects and behaviors in others. These patients don't show devaluation of objects as much as a terribly painful sense of abandonment by the objects. Schizoid personalities have a deep available potential for reconstructing meaningful emotional relationships once the defensive schizoid structure is resolved.

In short, the schizoid affect dissolution or dispersal can be differentiated from the usual defensive mechanisms of object relations of the paranoid-schizoid position. It is diagnosed through the typical development of emptiness in verbal transference communications and the central clarifying function of countertransference under these conditions that alerts the clinician to this specific constellation. Betty Joseph's (1989) stress on the importance of the analyst's diagnosis of the patient's efforts to influence the analyst, the patient's efforts to have the analyst perceive him or her in a certain way, may be helpful here. Schizoid patients unconsciously may attempt to convince the analyst that there is no emotional reality going on and that, under conditions of the present confusion, mutual withdrawal is the most reasonable reaction.

In summary, in all three cases the apparent content of transference developments had an unavailable or trivial quality that did not permit me to diagnose the presently dominant object relationship, while, to the contrary, the countertransference clearly indicated the differential quality of the underlying conflicts: the erotic-masochistic conflict of Jennifer, the passive aggressive dependency of Sarah, and the paranoid fear of attack in Robert. All three patients had been socially withdrawn, and even their withdrawal had a noncommunicative quality in Jennifer, showed indignant rejection in Sarah, and a expressed provocative readiness for a fight in Robert. The internal fantasy life of these patients, once it could be carefully reconstructed beyond the fragmentation of thinking processes, revealed Jennifer's erotic dreams, Sarah's indignant counter-rejection, and Robert's dangerous fantastical confrontations. Countertransference analysis permitted me to overcome the initial triviality of their verbal communication and gradually interpret within the transference the defensive schizoid structure—the discovery of the patients' deeper erotic, dependent, and aggressive conflicts.

Further Comments About Treatment

Should patients with schizoid personality disorders be analyzed or be treated with specialized psychoanalytic psychotherapies such as TFP for severe personality disorder? On the basis of the clinical experiences of the Personality Disorders Institute it seems that, given the secondary complications that the objective distance of treatment on the couch creates in terms of analyzing schizoid emptiness, the most severe cases that function on an overtly borderline level probably would respond best to TFP. In all cases, however, the treatment must include basic technical psychoanalytic conditions: the expectation that the patient carry out free associations and that the analyst carry out the interpretation of the developing transference manifestations from a position of technical neutrality, being particularly alert to countertransference developments. In all cases, then, interpretation, transference analysis, technical neutrality, and countertransference utilization are essential tools regardless of the treatment with TFP or standard analysis.

Transference analysis is made difficult over an extended early period because of its apparent absence of specificity given the dominant affect fragmentation. Interpretation must focus on the affective dispersal and correspondent cognitive fragmentation, with the help of the heightened awareness and use of countertransference activation. If countertransference alerts the therapist to subtle, fleeting affective developments in the hours, these may provide guidelines to the general affective dominance. The analysis of the analytic field in these cases—that is, the dominant implicit relationship that the total therapeutic situation determines for therapist and patient—may be particularly helpful. It is important to maintain technical neutrality, which may be made difficult by partial acting out of the countertransference once a more specific affective relationship emerges. As always, it is important to maintain the frame of the analytic setting and to be watchful for any significant denial of reality on the patient's part that may represent acting out of the emotionally dominant but fragmented affect.

During the early stages of the treatment, the striking absence of fantasy regarding central aspects of the patient's reality may guide one to what is being avoided. Life situations in terms of work and profession, love and sex, social life and creativity need to be explored carefully as indicators of what is being avoided in the transference. The patient's avoiding all sexual interactions and references may indicate an underlying extreme sadomasochistic aspect of early eroticism; the fact that the patient may chronically feel rejected by everybody and, enraged, reject the most important people in his or her life obviously indicates what the patient may be afraid will develop in the transference. A patient's dissociated hostility predicts the avoided violence in the sessions and the need to be prepared for such developments.

Above all, the frequent central dilemma of these patients—their search for intimacy as opposed to their panic over being invaded, swallowed up, or controlled sadistically—must be kept in mind and carefully explored in the transference. It is important to ventilate the patient's sense of brutal rejection as a consequence of minor disappointments with attitudes of the therapist or of being sadistically intruded upon because the therapist raises a clarifying question. These are frequent challenges in dealing with the basic dilemma of these patients. It is important that the therapist be ready to acknowledge errors or mistakes in his or her interventions when the patient has the sense of being submitted to a dogmatic brainwashing. It may be helpful to clarify to the patient that, in effect, one is interested in understanding what is going on in the patient but that one respects the patient's deep mistrust in that interest and that one is aware of the patient's experience of being ignored in the process.

I trust that what has been said thus far illustrates the contrast with cases of narcissistic grandiosity, in which therapist and patient exchange their roles, alternating between grandiose and humiliated aspects of the patient's self in the transference. I trust that these cases also illustrate a contrast to a symbiotic intolerance of triangulation, in which the patient insists on the importance that the therapist agree with him or her totally and have no ideas that are different or independent from the patient's thinking. The schizoid transferences clearly show the difference from the splitting phenomena that are part of the paranoid-schizoid position of borderline personality organization in analytic treatment and, of course, are very different from the "ordinary" intense development of neurotic transference relationships in which the patient identifies with an infantile aspect of the self and projects the corresponding representation of parental objects onto the analyst.

References

Akhtar S: Broken Structures. Northvale, NJ, Jason Aronson, 1992, pp 123–147

American Psychiatric Association: Diagnostic and Statistical Manual of Mental Disorders, 5th Edition. Arlington, VA, American Psychiatric Association, 2013, pp 652–655

Fairbairn W: Object-Relations Theory of the Personality. New York, Basic Books, 1954

Guntrip H: Personality Structure and Human Interaction. London, Hogarth, 1961

Guntrip H: Schizoid Phenomena, Object-Relations and the Self. New York, International Universities Press, 1969

Joseph B: Object relations in clinical practice, in Psychic Equilibrium and Psychic Change. Edited by Feldman M, Spillius EB. London, Routledge, 1989, pp 203–215

Kernberg OF: Identity: recent findings and clinical implications, in The Inseparable Nature of Love and Aggression: Clinical and Theoretical Perspectives. Washington, DC, American Psychiatric Publishing, 2011, pp 3–30

Klein M: Notes on some schizoid mechanisms. Int J Psychoanal 27:99–110, 1946

Klein M: Some theoretical conclusions regarding the emotional life of the infant, in Developments in Psychoanalysis. Edited by Klein M, Heimann P, Isaacs S, Riviere J. London, Hogarth, 1952, pp 198–236

Klein M: On the development of mental functioning. Int J Psychoanal 39:84–90, 1958

McWilliams N: Psychoanalytic Diagnosis, 2nd Edition. New York, Guilford, 2011, pp 196–213

Yeomans FE, Clarkin JF, Kernberg OF: Transference Focused Psychotherapy for Borderline Personality Disorder. Washington, DC, American Psychiatric Publishing, 2015

CHAPTER 8

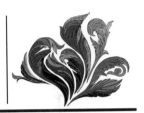

Psychotic Personality Structure

To begin, I am limiting the terms *psychosis* and *psychotic functioning* to the behavioral manifestations of patients who have lost the capacity of reality testing. Assessing the presence or absence of reality testing permits the differentiation of psychotic from non-psychotic functioning. Reality testing consists of the ability to differentiate self from non-self, intrapsychic from external origin of stimuli, and the capacity to maintain empathy with ordinary social criteria for reality (Kernberg 1984; Oyebode 2018). Reality testing can be assessed in a structural diagnostic interview and, in fact, in any careful mental status interview, by focusing at some point on what seems most strange or inappropriate in a patient's behavior, affect, thought content, or organization of language. The patient's capacity to empathize with the therapist's tactful observation of what seems strange in the patient's communication permits us to assess the patient's reality testing. Obviously, the loss of reality testing is most clearly evident in the presence of true hallucinations, delusions, and in behaviors that reflect a more or less subtle or even gross distortion in what would ordinarily be expected normal behavior in a diagnostic interview.

Reality testing has to be differentiated from the experience of reality and from the relationship to reality. The experience of reality may vary widely under the impact of affect activation and the development of more permanent and generalized moods, as well as under the influence of alcohol or drugs. Alteration in the experience of reality does not necessarily coincide with loss of reality testing, and often individuals who experience such change in their experience of reality can evaluate this very realistically. The relationship with reality, in turn, may become inappropriate, particularly under the effect of peak affect states. In moments of intensely emotional experience, not only patients but all people may behave crazily, acting, talking, and thinking inappropriately. However, when reality testing is maintained, the patient may be fully aware of the inappropriate nature of his behavior once the affect has returned to normal. Under conditions of a bipolar illness, with long-term severe abnormalities in affect experience and expression, reality testing may be affected, signaling the psychotic nature of manic and severe depressive conditions.

From the viewpoint of psychoanalytic object relations theory, the loss of reality testing implies a loss of the boundaries between self and object representations, the incapacity to differentiate the self-experience from the experience of the other, a related incapacity to assess the unrealistic aspect of behavioral manifestations in the interaction of self with others, and the resulting confusion in the assessment of the actual interpersonal situation. The clinical experience with patients who present severe personality disorders and a related predominance of primitive defense operations is reflected in inappropriate interpersonal behaviors as well as inappropriate affect activation and misinterpretations of the immediate interaction. However, in such cases, the patient maintains a clear sense of difference between self and other, even if there evolves a rapid exchange of their experienced respective roles. The interaction is open to a therapist's realistic assessment. When the nature of the distorted interaction is rationally reframed in the light of obvious social reality, borderline patients are capable of recognizing their distorted reactions. In other words, under the effect of interpretation, the patient is able to contain the unrealistic transferential experience that is being examined and explore it from the viewpoint of appropriate reality testing.

Melanie Klein (1946) described the primitive mechanisms that characterize the paranoid-schizoid position and the depressive position, and convincingly, I believe, proposed that the paranoid-schizoid mechanisms were the essential defensive operations of schizophrenia, while manic-depressive illness was dominated by the defensive mechanisms of the depressive position and the manic defenses related to them. At the same time, she made it clear that she did not assume that infants normally would develop these psychotic syndromes, thus differentiating the clinical conditions of schizophrenia and manic-depressive illness from the primitive mechanisms dominant in them. In fact, it is an important basic psychodynamic finding, I believe, that in both psychotic and borderline personality organization, there is a predominance of these primitive defensive operations, particularly centered on splitting and projective identification, in contrast to higher-level defensive operations centered on repression in neurotic personality organization (Kernberg 2004). However, the predominance of primitive mechanisms does not coincide with psychotic personality organization. It is reality testing that determines that differentiation, not the predominance of primitive defensive operations. Permanent loss of reality testing is a reflection of refusion of self and object representations.

The general assumption of object relations theory is that the fundamental organization of the mind is determined by the development of primary dyadic units of internalized representations of self interacting with representations of others under the impact of dominant or peak affect states that reflect both the primary motivational features and the nature of all internalized interpersonal interactions from birth on. The combined integrated motivational pressure of positive affect systems constitutes libido as the superordinate drive, and the integration of negative affect systems constitutes aggression as the superordinate drive (Kernberg 1992). The gradual integration of the concept of the self, both into a libidinally integrated, ideal concept of self and into a split-off concept of the bad, unacceptable, dangerous part of the self under the dominance of aggression, with parallel developments of such respectively good and bad representations of dominant internalized objects, constitutes an early level of development. Fixation at this developmental stage—with a permanent split of self-representations into idealized and persecuted or devalued ones and a parallel split of object representations into idealized and persecutory ones—determines the syndrome of identity diffusion characteristic of borderline personality organization.

Eventually, under the dominance of the depressive position, an integrated concept of self that combines good and bad aspects consolidates and overcomes the earliest dichotomy of the paranoid-schizoid position. An integrated concept of the self- and integrated representations of significant others, both good and bad, determines identity integration characteristic of neurotic personality organization and normality (Kemberg and Caligor 2005) (see Table 8–1). Melanie Klein stressed that the intensity of inborn aggression, what we might now call the intensity of negative affect dispositions, is the main etiological disposition that determines the degree of severity of pathology at the psychotic or borderline level.

The original observation that loss of reality testing reflected a refusion of the representations of self with the representations of others was provided in Edith Jacobson's (1971) study of neurotic, borderline, and

Table 8–1. Personality structure, transference, and outcome

Personality organization	Structural interview	Psychoanalysis or TFP	Outcome
Neurotic	Normal identity; excellent reality testing	No psychotic regression	Characterological improvement
Borderline	Identity diffusion; reality testing maintained but restricted	Possible psychotic transference	Probable resolution of identity diffusion and excellent reality testing
Psychotic	Identity diffusion; loss of reality testing	Possible transference psychosis	Slow reduction of transference psychosis with treatment suspension
Chronic schizophrenia	Overtly positive and negative psychotic symptoms	Permanent psychotic transference and psychotic functioning in social reality	Improvement in social functioning

Source. From Kernberg OF: "Psychotic Personality Structure." *Psychodynamic Psychiatry* 47(4):353–372, 2019. Copyright © 2019 Guilford Press. Reprinted with permission of Guilford Press.

psychotic depression. She observed that primitive defensive operations disorganized the behavior in the transference manifestations of borderline patients but did not affect their reality testing, while the same primitive defensive operations, under conditions of psychotic depression, did profoundly affect reality testing. Jacobson found that, in psychotic depression, refusion between self-representations and object representations evolved in the area of actual interactions between self and other and in the area of idealized representations of self and other; in other words, in the ego as well as in the ego ideal, the idealizing aspect of the superego. Further, insofar as in psychotic depression the refusion between self- and object representations occurred within both ego and superego while boundaries between superego and ego were still maintained, patients were still able to differentiate themselves and their experience clearly from the analyst, while, under the effect of projective and introjective processes, the experience of self and other were severely distorted. It was only under conditions of schizophrenic illness, where refusion of self- and object representations were general, that a permanent disorganization evolved and the typical symptoms of chronic hallucinations, delusions, and disorganized thinking and behavior prevailed.

Jacobson pointed to the extremely primitive nature of refusion between ideal self and ideal object representations as the ultimate defense against aggression, leading, in turn, to the corresponding lack of differentiation between bad self- and bad object representations that determines the structure of psychotic states. That double refusion, in turn, prevents not only a clear differentiation of external reality and the patient's interactions with it, but by its combination with introjective and projective processes, a confusion between ideal and persecutory conditions evolves, the confusional states between what is good and what is bad that Rosenfeld (1950) described in chronic schizophrenic patients.

In agreement with Edith Jacobson, I believe that psychotic personality organization corresponds to an intrapsychic predominance of refusion of self- and object representations in the area of idealized as well as persecutory internalized object relations, clinically reflected in loss of reality testing. But temporary loss of reality testing also may evolve in borderline personality organization, with different features, as we shall see.

Here, I would consider the implications stemming from the neurobiological research on the etiology and neuropathological aspects of schizophrenia. Research on the etiology of schizophrenia has pointed to the combination of genetic disposition and environmental causes of this illness. The genetic disposition may have a major influence on the pathology of brain structures characteristic of schizophrenia that include the thinning of the prefrontal cortex and of the parietal and temporal cortex, particular abnormalities of the dorsolateral area of the prefrontal cortex, the amygdala, the hippocampus, and the speech centers (Hyman and Cohen 2013). Each of these areas is crucially involved with the registration of affectively invested self- and object representations (Förstl 2012).

The interrelationship between the amygdala and the prefrontal cortex controls and cognitively contextualizes affect activation; the dorsolateral aspect of the prefrontal cortex is related to working memory and to early integration of the perception of others, while the ventromedial part of the prefrontal cortex is intimately related with the development of the experience of self (Förstl et al. 2006). My point is that the neurobiological predisposition to schizophrenia may particularly affect the structures related to setting up the internal world of differentiated representations of self and others, the cortical control and contextualization of affective experience, thus contributing to affective memory structures that interfere with the normal contextualization of affect and self- and object differentiations (Hart 2008).

Concretely, mother's ability to contain the infant's projection (and reintrojection) of intolerable negative affect states would be severely interfered with by such a pathological neurobiological structure. This may lead to extreme negative affect states and terrors that predispose to the equally extreme defensive effort to refuse positive self- and object representations and, secondarily, negative ones as well. In contrast, given the normal potential for development of short-time affective memory guaranteed by normal prefrontal and limbic structures, the safe differentiation between self- and object representations both in the idealized and persecutory regions of the mind may take place. From here, development may proceed toward the fixation of a permanent state of identity diffusion typical of borderline personality organization or, under more favorable circumstances, the establishment of normal identity integration with the development of the depressive position and the establishment of neurotic personality organization or, simply, normality.

The lack of boundaries between self- and object representations represents a devastating loss of the capacity to accurately assess reality, and it may be relevant that of the three major symptom groups of schizophrenia—namely 1) positive symptoms (hallucinations, delusions), 2) negative symptoms (social withdrawal, isolation, amotivational relations to the social world), and 3) general disorganization characterized by thought disorder, peculiarities of language, and cognitive deterioration—the last one may persist even when positive and negative symptoms improve with treatment and result in better social functioning.

In addition to the abnormality of certain brain structures, the abnormality of some key neurotransmitters also may be involved in the alteration of the perception of reality in schizophrenia. One important aspect of these abnormalities, an abnormal dominance of dopaminergic functions, may be related to excessive activity of the affective "seeking system" that motivates exploration of reality, leading to an excessive stimulus input that interferes with the assessment of reality under the condition of activation of other affective systems (Panksepp and Biven 2012). Effective psychopharmacological treatment of schizophrenia reduces dopaminergic functions. Yet psychopharmacological treatment does not affect the cognitive disorganization when it is prominent, and it is possible to diagnose residual alterations of reality testing in the clinical examination of patients during periods of latency of illness (Hyman and Cohen 2013).

At the same time, it is emerging that psychotherapeutic treatment continues to have an important role, particularly for patients who, as Michael Stone (1993) has concluded, present with a combination of a significant degree of functioning affect differentiation, maintenance of a high intellectual level, and lack of antisocial features. Psychotherapy seems particularly relevant for patients whose response to psychopharmacological treatment has been limited and who have not been able to fully recover reality testing.

Many chronic schizophrenic patients are able to maintain ordinary relations with reality other than that involving intimate relations with significant others or experience the condition of what has been called "benign delusional syndromes." Many such patients understand that their reality is different from others and learn to mask their delusions in order to appear more normal than they feel. A modality of psychoanalytic psychotherapy that respects such limited persistence of residual phenomena of benign delusions may permit patients to function socially in an acceptable way.

Elizabeth Spillius and colleagues (2011) point to the gradual disillusionment with and abandonment of major Kleinian efforts in the therapy of schizophrenia, with the exception of analysts connected with psychiatric institutions who continue to provide various types of psychoanalytic psychotherapy to some of these patients. New methods of these psychoanalytic psychotherapies have been developed in recent years, but this is not the subject of the present article (Garrett 2019).

There are extreme psychological and social conditions under which reality testing may be lost, including severely pathological sadomasochistic relations of intimate couples who present mutual reinforcement of primitive defensive operations, such as in cases of *folie à deux* (shared psychotic disorder). There are certain regressive large group consolidations under extreme social deprivation or isolation—such as religious cults, where similar phenomena of collective loss of reality testing may take place. But there are also experiences in which momentary loss of differentiation between self and others occurs, such as under some conditions of intense orgastic experiences of a couple intimately related or of an extremely hateful momentary merger between torturer and his victim. These latter conditions have a momentary quality that does not reflect a psychotic personality organization.

Clinically, patients who only under intense, intimate interactions manifest loss of reality testing and who are able, most of the time, to function within normal social boundaries are probably the most prevalent cases of "psychotic personality organization" without manifest psychosis. These patients can be diagnosed using structural interviews and may be prone to psychotic regression under the intensity of a psychoanalytic exploration, which may then expand into a general, chronic psychotic condition. This differentiates them sharply from the opposite development in cases with borderline personality organization, where a psychoanalytic approach improves the relationship with reality in the context of the resolution of primitive defensive operations and of the massive splitting between idealized and paranoid experiences.

Clinically, the most frequent syndromes in which we find psychotic personality organization other than schizophrenia are major depression with psychosis, manic syndromes, paranoid psychoses, and drug-induced psychosis. The development of the psychotic regression in borderline personality organization typically manifest in psychotic transferences differs from the chronic psychotic regression of patients with psychotic personality organization who were not clinically psychotic before psychoanalytic exploration. These latter cases include many patients with hypochondriasis, body dysmorphic syndromes, morbid jealousy, and some severe cases of anorexia nervosa (Oyebode 2018). Psychosis induced in the course of transference regression that then becomes chronic should be differentiated from "psychotic transferences" that express transference regression, remain limited to the transference, and can be interpretatively resolved.

In each of these conditions—psychotic personality organization, actual psychosis, and transference psychosis—there is a predominance of primitive defensive operations similar to borderline personality organization and, we might add, a prevalence of primitive preoedipal and oedipal conflicts under the dominance of aggression and regressive negative affect states. And, of course, the universality of these unconscious conflicts is reflected in neurotic personality organization as well and in the analytic exploration of group processes, couples treatment, and complex posttraumatic conditions. In what follows, I briefly present illustrations of some frequent clinical conditions.

The clinical material presented reflects both the essential aspects of the psychopathology of these cases and the utilization of psychodynamic constructs outlined in this article. These cases have been selected for presentation from clinical work carried out with patients that I myself have treated, others that I supervised, and others treated at different psychiatric hospitals where I worked over the years.

CASE 1: THE CASE OF ANNA[1]

Anna was a woman in her middle twenties who suffered from a paranoid schizophrenic illness since late adolescence and who had been treated with several atypical antipsychotic drugs. She was able to func-

---

[1] Names and details have been changed to protect patient privacy.

tion in simple daily tasks but lived an isolated existence, with chronic hallucinations involving neighbors who, she thought, wanted to influence her by electronic rays sent throughout the building in which she lived. Her past history reflected a benign, somewhat distant, and permissive father and a very dominant, controlling mother who gave Anna the impression throughout her childhood that "mother knew it all." The patient's experience of the all-powerful mother was displaced onto the neighbors, who now had the power to control her by means of electricity sent through the walls of her apartment. The patient felt that to move to a new place was useless in terms of protecting her against this ongoing neighbors' conspiracy. In the course of her psychoanalytic psychotherapy, she gradually established a dependent relation with me.

She perceived me as someone with a social background and political views similar to her own. Any efforts to analyze her experiences with the potential persecutors in terms of a maternal transference led to intense anxiety and disorganization that was reduced as soon as the subject changed to what she felt indicated her and my common interests. Over a period of many months, she was able to share with me all the issues for which she could be criticized by these imaginary persecutory neighbors as well as her guilt feelings over masturbatory activities that contained fantasies about sexual relations between her parents, fantasies that were frightening and exciting at the same time. Anna had relationships with boyfriends in early adolescence that always came to a sudden end when they attempted to achieve a more intimate sexual relationship with her. During the course of Anna's illness, her mother died, leading to an intensification of the psychotic symptoms that had brought her into treatment. The combination of resentment about her mother's control over her and guilt feelings about her rebellious opposition to her mother in her early sexual behavior was an important subject of the early stages of treatment. But any effort to explore her subtle seductive attitude in the transference and her unassailable conviction that we were both united in adopting her political and social thinking proved highly resistant.

I finally accepted an apparent agreement on common philosophical views as the justification for her intense gratification with our sessions, while the assurance that nothing sexual could emerge in them led to her trusting me with her convictions about her neighbors penetrating her with electricity and sexual fantasies. I was able gradually to point out 1) that her capacity to experience the critical attitude toward her through the walls of the building reflected a unique refinement of her sensitivity to criticism derived from the experience with her mother, a refined receptiveness that was really not available to anybody else; and 2) that therefore the people that apparently were criticizing her could not harm her in reality, because they did not have the subtlety of perception of her and her mother that might affect her. This complicated kind of reasoning permitted her to accept the fact that she had these experiences without having to take them seriously, because, in her perception of reality, all the potentially critical others really could not reach her. The alliance with me as the one who acknowledged her implicit superiority and thus protected her against the fear of the influences throughout the walls permitted her to

establish an equilibrium that resulted in an increase of her social functioning, her work capacity, and relationships with people on a friendly
basis that was satisfying to her in her daily life, while the psychotic state
resisted unchanged. Here, a fused ideal self- and object representation
protected her efficiently against the persecutory fused rebellious self/
sadistic mother, in an obvious psychotic personality organization.

CASE 2: THE CASE OF ELIZABETH

Elizabeth, a woman in her early twenties, presented an agitated, disorganized acute schizophrenic illness, with chaotic sexual and persecutory
delusions and hallucinations and a fixed idea that she had been selected
by the devil to be his mistress as well as his leading mistress/prostitute
who could seduce all the men in the world. She also had fantasies that
her genitals had been hyperstimulated and destroyed. She masturbated
almost continuously while smelling her fingers, in the process tearing off
all clothing and having to be kept in a locked observation room. This was
before major antipsychotic medication was available, and I attempted to
treat her analytically.

It was an intense 9-month treatment, in the course of which the patient was able to improve. The outcome may reflect the positive prognosis
of a first psychotic episode, but I believe it was significantly influenced
by the analytic approach I followed. As I saw the patient daily in her
padded cell, naked and masturbating, I was struck by the absence of any
erotic reaction towards her. I was aware of some fear of the possibility
that she might assault me. After seeing her five times a week for several
weeks, during which she virtually refused to acknowledge my presence,
she began to take notice of me. She started to interrogate me about the
way I was dressed, whom I represented, whether I was spying on her,
and let me know that she had an intimate relation with the devil. She told
me I was an uninteresting bystander to the secure and exciting world
she shared with the devil, from which I was excluded. This long interim,
with a strong derogatory quality, shifted eventually into an intense challenge about where I stood regarding religion, God, and the devil. All the
while, despite my presence and the constant observation of the nursing
staff during our sessions, she continued masturbating. Our sessions
then evolved into an affectively intense situation in which she started
accusing me of being the devil and of wanting to seduce her, while at the
same time telling me that she was the devil and was going to seduce me.

The verbal communication became extremely confusing: We were
each the devil and, at the same time, each the victim of the other. There
were moments when she triumphantly noted that I looked frightened
and disturbed, confused about what to say, and, in fact, I was feeling
that way. My interventions then shifted to pointing out that there was a
dialogue going on between her and the devil in which it wasn't clear
whether she was trying to seduce the devil or the devil was trying to seduce her. And there were the questions we were both struggling with:
Was I the devil or his victim, or to what extent was I both? At each point
I attempted to stress that, in clarifying who I was, I was also trying to
clarify that I was a different person from her.

Technically speaking, it was what Harold Searles (1965) would have called a *symbiotic relationship* and what I would describe as a *transference psychosis* in which there was no differentiation between her representation of self and object. She viewed me as both at the same time, or as interchanging roles between these two participants, a seducing devil and his victim.

In a later stage of this treatment, approximately 6 months since the start, two new developments took place. She began to look at me "from a distance" or rather as if, at that point, she really experienced herself as a different person from me. As the symbiotic transference decreased, I, for the first time, experienced erotic feelings toward the frank sexuality she exhibited in my presence. As she differentiated herself from me, she became acutely seductive, and my countertransference became problematically erotic. Sensing my attempt to distance myself from her, she requested to be dressed in clothes. Seeing her in appropriate dress came as quite a shock. That initiated the final months of the treatment, when she faced the fact that we would have to separate because my time at the hospital was coming to an end. The last few months were a period of sadness and anxiety over our separation and her transfer to another psychotherapist. At that point, she was no longer psychotic but rather felt depressed, frightened, and worried about the severe psychotic experience she had lived through.

CASE 3: THE CASE OF PAUL

The treatment of Paul, a third schizophrenic patient, was of very brief duration. During his diagnostic evaluation, I had a sense of a strange attitude, his conviction of his being particularly sensitive to religious reality, which I found problematic. However, his statement was sufficiently harmonious with his religious background from a strictly traditional Southern Baptist environment, and his excessive concerns about religion seemed socially understandable. Two or three weeks after starting psychoanalytic treatment, during which he expressed that I would not be able to accompany him at the level at which he was perceiving human reality, it turned out he had a deep conviction that he was really Jesus Christ and was trying to live up to his mission to save the world. In the course of two or three treatment sessions, it became evident that his religious concerns had transformed themselves into an acute delusional conviction. He said I had contributed to clarifying his thoughts.

When I consulted with an experienced colleague, he confirmed that Paul was having an acute psychotic break. Paul's condition worsened in the next several weeks, and he was hospitalized with a diagnosis of an acute paranoid psychosis. Eventually, during his extended hospitalization, he was diagnosed with schizophrenia and responded positively to psychopharmacological treatment. After his discharge, it was recommended that he enter into psychotherapeutic rather than psychoanalytic treatment. The treatment I initiated was standard psychoanalysis, four weekly sessions. This treatment was interrupted after 6 weeks for the reasons mentioned before.

These three cases clearly were schizophrenic patients. The first case, Anna, was treated with a mostly supportive approach, psychoanalytically oriented, in contrast to the second case, Elizabeth, who was treated with a psychoanalytic approach following Searles's orientation. Harold Searles (1965) describes psychoanalytic psychotherapy with schizophrenia patients as evolving in several stages—first, a phase of lack of interactive contact, followed by an intense symbiotic phase, the resolution of which would lead to conflicts of separation and individualization and hopefully, eventually, to new integration and identity formation. Paul's brief treatment was the initiation of psychoanalysis.

Additional Cases

The cases that follow represent non-psychotic patients who develop a transference psychosis—that is, a loss of reality testing during the course of psychoanalytic treatment—that evolves into a full-blown psychotic syndrome which may be resolved with the end of the psychoanalytic approach but may persist for an extended time. In other words, it is a psychosis that clearly evolves from transference developments but is not resolvable by means of transference interpretation.

LUIS

The first patient, Luis, was a man in his thirties, with a paranoid personality and strongly narcissistic and schizoid features. He underwent psychoanalysis with an advanced psychoanalytic candidate. In the course of treatment, he evinced intense oedipal conflicts with his father. In fact, during childhood and adolescence, his father had suspected him of all kinds of sexual behavior for which he would be severely punished. These experiences were linked to a hidden rebellious attitude, with intense hatred of both his father and his mother, who he felt supported his father in his persecutory and punishing attitude towards him.

At one point, Luis developed intense resentment of the analyst, whom he experienced in the transference as making fun of him, enjoying torturing him, and being dishonest with him. Gradually, Luis developed the fantasy that the analyst was attempting to have a sexual affair with his mother, and he connected a number of coincidences between the analyst's absences and his mother's absences from town; at the same time, he developed the fantasy that his mother and the analyst were carrying on their affair in a different city. At first, the analyst interpreted this as an oedipal fantasy, but over the course of the sessions, this became more and more of a conviction, to the point where Luis came to a session with a gun and threatened to shoot the analyst if he refused to stop the affair. At that point, the analyst stopped treatment and referred the patient to another therapist. We later learned that in the course of supportive, reality-oriented treatment over a period of several months, Luis gradually abandoned the idea that his previous analyst had had an affair with his mother and remained functioning at a nonpsychotic level.

MARIA

A similar case is that of Maria, a patient with hypochondriasis, who started in transference-focused psychotherapy (TFP) with an experienced therapist in the course of which her hypochondriacal symptoms gradually became transformed into a transference psychosis. The patient presented chronic hypochondriacal symptoms involving her teeth, dental pain that could not be resolved by various dental treatments. In entering psychotherapy, her concern about her dental pain and the fact that nobody was able to fix it became a dominant theme: her resentment about the incompetence and grandiosity of dentists and physicians in general. Over the course of several months, she went into treatment with several dentists and, gradually, as these dentists contacted each other and reached the conclusion that they couldn't find the cause for her symptoms, she developed the delusion that the dentists were united in a conspiracy to mistreat her and give her false hope while being in agreement to prolong her suffering. The delusion about the conspiracy of dentists then extended to the dental organization of the state, and finally evolved into the delusion that the therapist was in cahoots with the dental organization and was supporting them by attempting to convince her that there was no such conspiracy. She developed the delusion that the therapist was contributing to the conspiracy in order to make her a victim of permanent dental pain. She blamed the dental organization for sending her from one dentist to another without ever helping her to get better. The intensity of her resentment and hatred of the therapist could not be dealt with by efforts to deal interpretively with this transference development, and the therapist decided to stop the treatment at that point. He referred her to another therapist, who carried out a supportive psychotherapy combined with antidepressant medication to reduce her anxiety and convinced her to consult a chronic pain management clinic, while the conviction about the conspiracy participation by the therapist gradually decreased.

These are cases of true transference psychosis that have to be differentiated from cases in which psychotic transferences develop but may be treated in the transference and do not expand into the external life and total life experiences of the patient. In all of these cases, reality testing was lost, but while we may assume a psychotic personality organization in the cases I have mentioned so far, this is not the case of the patients that follow.

SALLY

Sally was a patient in her early twenties with a borderline personality disorder, severe narcissistic features, chronic characterological depression, frequent and severe suicidal attempts, temper tantrums that would lead to suicide attempts, drug abuse, and sexual promiscuity. This patient had been brought up and severely mistreated by an aunt during her childhood, to the extent that she didn't participate in physical exercise at school in order to conceal the black and blue bruises all over her body. In treatment, she threatened, if not responded to immediately, to attempt suicide, and three therapists ended treatment because they could not tolerate her constant threat of suicidal behavior that was followed, in effect, by severe suicide attempts.

In TFP treatment with me, we set limits on how to manage her chronic suicidality as well as her between-session phone contacts. I explained our usual approach to the control of treatment-threatening, acting-out behavior by pointing out that if she had symptoms she could not control, she was free to go to the emergency room of a psychiatric hospital but not to contact me between sessions. If she could control whatever was threatening her without having to go to an emergency room, we could discuss it in the following session. I told her that I would accept her telephone calls for unforeseen, unexpected emergencies only, but not for issues regarding what we had previously discussed. Suicidal impulses represented an issue she knew exactly how to handle. I made it clear that I would not respond to a phone call dealing with suicidal fears and that if she repeated these calls, I would successively not take calls for a week or, if her behavior continued unchanged, for a month, for a year, and even, if necessary, for the entire treatment! The calls stopped when she became aware that I did not answer them for a period of a month.

But then Sally developed the fantasy that one of my secretaries was secretly calling her, remaining silent or murmuring insults into her phone. Sally occasionally received what were considered erroneous calls, and she developed the fantasy that in all those cases there was a derogatory attitude expressed towards her. Finally, she became convinced she was being called persistently at home by my secretary, whom she wanted me to dismiss, threatening to report me to the state medical board for harassment if I didn't take that action. She became extremely afraid and enraged about these assumed telephone attacks.

I interpreted those fears as hallucinatory experiences and delusion formations as part of the transference regression in which a projection of her sadistic and omnipotent controlling behavior was dominant. The patient felt that, through my secretary, I was secretly attempting to torture her and disorganize her life, as her aunt had done in the past. Systematic interpretation of this transference, without at any point reassuring her that her interpretation of the calls was an error and without trying to rationally convince her that I would not tolerate such behavior by my secretary, permitted us to resolve this conviction that, at one point, had threatened potential termination of the treatment with me and the search for another therapist to escape my supposed sadistic behavior.

I utilized the method of interpretation of "incompatible realities" that we found very helpful in cases of psychotic transferences in our work at the Personalities Disorders Institute at Cornell. The intervention consists of pointing out to the patient that we have a completely different view of whatever he or she is convinced of at that moment, without trying to impose our view. The question is whether the view of the therapist is dishonest, whether the therapist basically knows that the patient is right and only pretends to think differently for whatever reason, or whether the therapist is honest in his radically opposite view. Does the therapist honestly believe in something totally opposite to the patient's thinking, something that, in fact, is totally incompatible with the patient's thinking?

Here, we reach the conclusion that one of the two, the patient or the therapist, must be out of reality, without it being possible to decide who is in step with reality and who is out of it, and that both must accept that a psychotic reality is evolving that affects both of them and needs to be examined on its own merits. By establishing a boundary around the psychotic conviction, we can analyze the basic situation in the transference and resolve it in the transference rather than in a discussion of who is right and who is out of reality. It is an effective way of transference interpretation under conditions of psychotic transference regression, very effective with severe psychotic regression that may occur in the treatment of borderline personality organization but typically ineffective in patients with a psychotic personality organization.

MICHAEL

A similar case presenting a psychotic transference is that of Michael, a physician in his forties with a severe narcissistic personality disorder and sexual promiscuity. In the course of his treatment, after 4 years of analysis and when primitive oedipal problems became dominant in the transference, Michael was pursuing a nurse who mentioned at one point that she knew me. He was confident he could get her to have sex with him, and when she refused, his reaction was intense rage not only with her but mostly with me as well. He developed the delusion that I had forbidden all the nurses in all the services of the medical university to get involved with him sexually.

He appeared the next morning for a session in full rage, ready to beat me up. Only after I obtained his assurance that he would not attempt to physically attack me was he willing to talk about this situation. In using the technique of incompatible realities, I pointed out to him that I thought his assumption that I had forbidden all the nurses to go to bed with him seemed completely crazy to me. Although I was not attempting to convince him of my view, I wanted him to understand that we had completely incompatible views and, as I pointed out, that at this point one of us must be crazy. My first suggestion to him was the possibility that I might be lying to him, denying my instructions to the nurses. Interestingly enough, he didn't think I had overtly instructed the nurses to reject him but rather that I might have given secret signals, perhaps even unknowingly, using behavioral gestures indicating to the entire nursing profession that he was not a man anybody should go to bed with. I categorically expressed my disagreement. So, at the end, it became clear that this was a psychotic situation involving us. I pointed out that its content was that of a powerful man making sure that another man, who depended on him, was being prevented from sexually seducing women, as if he were being symbolically castrated. That observation led to a sudden memory by the patient, from when he was 6 or 7 years old, of his father cutting the vocal cords of their two dogs because they were barking all night—a violent gesture from a violent father who had terrorized him throughout his childhood—and that now emerged with an intensity that made it an immediate reality. The delusional conviction became a transference repetition of the resentment and fear linked to the conflict with his father.

I would add to these clinical illustrations some general considerations regarding the analytic diagnosis and management of psychotic conditions in which reality testing is lost. Not all of these conditions reflect a psychotic organization of the personality, and I question the concept that there is always a psychotic personality underlying various degrees of transference regression. If the basic personality structure is characterized by a dominance of refusion between self- and object representations—even if such a refusion occurs only under conditions of intense affect activation in intimate personal situations—the term *psychotic personality organization* is warranted, even with patients who are not clinically psychotic at that point. Psychotic personality organization may be diagnosed in a careful mental status examination where loss of reality testing can be elicited.

Cases with such psychotic personality organization who are not clinically psychotic may be treated by various approaches depending on their symptomatology. However, it is unclear whether they can be treated with psychoanalysis proper, because the regressive effects of psychoanalysis proper may trigger a transference psychosis that may not be resolved in psychoanalytic treatment, whether it be psychoanalysis or TFP. At the same time, if the patient is clearly psychotic, psychoanalytic psychotherapy may be helpful as long it is clear that the technical approach is different from standard psychoanalysis and from TFP. The cases of Anna and Elizabeth illustrate this approach. The present article did not intend to spell out such an approach in more detail. There are cases in which acknowledging the risk of a transference psychosis may still warrant a psychoanalytic approach, probably TFP rather than standard psychoanalysis, if one is prepared to shift into a supportive direction in case it seems that a chronic psychotic condition may be triggered.

Patients with borderline personality organization have a clear indication for TFP, but there may be cases that can be treated with standard psychoanalysis using some TFP techniques, such as the treatment of incompatible reality. The cases of Sally and Michael illustrate this approach. The development of a psychotic transference may be managed effectively with psychoanalytic techniques, and there is no reason to shift the approach to a patient who is being treated analytically. A psychotic transference can be differentiated from a transference psychosis in the limitation of hallucinatory and delusional contents to the transference situation, while a transference psychosis is characterized by the expansion of psychotic symptoms to the entire life situation of the patient. The cases of Luis and Maria illustrate this development.

One important precondition for deciding what treatment approach might be most helpful is a careful diagnostic evaluation. Unfortunately, there is still a traditional tendency of many psychoanalysts to trust in the development of an adequate diagnostic understanding over the course of treatment rather than beginning from a diagnostic formulation that informs the treatment. That leads to many therapeutic disappointments and, I believe, is not an appropriate, responsible therapeutic approach. All patients should be carefully evaluated initially in terms of their predominant personality organization to differentiate the severity of pathology and, if the question emerges, to carefully diagnose reality testing. In all cases, the analysis of primitive defensive operations and the analysis of pre-oedipal and oedipal conflicts activated in the context of such defensive operations need to be fully explored in psychoanalytic treatments, and each patient will be different from all others in this regard.

Everything I have said so far implies the usefulness of structural analysis of the personality in terms of a general psychoanalytic strategy, but there is no further relevance of such structural considerations in terms of the approach to each patient in each session once the nature of the treatment has been decided upon. We have available important clinical research about the effects of different psychoanalytic approaches, and we should be able to creatively use various combinations of these psychoanalytic instruments, in contrast to assuming that all patients should be treated with the same approach. There are patients who get worse with psychoanalytic treatment, and there are patients who can be helped with techniques that use psychoanalytic instruments in new and creative ways.

To conclude, the diagnosis of psychotic personality organization should be reserved for patients who suffer from significant primary fusion or refusion of self- and object representations, particularly under intense affect activation, reflected in clinical psychosis and transference psychosis.

Diagnostically, these patients usually reveal loss of reality testing in structural diagnostic interviews but may only regress into psychosis in treatments that evolve into transference psychosis. Psychotic transferences may emerge in psychotic and borderline personality organization but are typically restricted to the transference in borderline patients, where they may be analytically resolved with particular psychoanalytic methods. Psychotic transferences that evolve into transference psychosis, with extension into the patient's total life situation, are typically linked to psychotic personality organization and signal a potential limitation to psychoanalytic treatment. Table 8–1 summarizes the overall relationship between personality organization, structural interview, and psychotic developments in the transference and in the patient's life.

References

Förstl H: Theory of Mind, 2nd Edition. Heidelberg, Springer Medizin, 2012

Förstl H, Hautzinger M, Roth G: Neurobiologie Psychischer Stöungen. Heidelberg, Springer Medizin, 2006

Garrett M: Psychotherapy of Psychosis. New York, Guilford, 2019

Hart S: Brain, Attachment, Personality. London, Karnac, 2008

Hyman SE, Cohen JD: Disorders of thought and volition: schizophrenia, in Principles of Neural Sciences, 5th Edition. Edited by Kandel ER, Schwartz JH, Jenal TM, et al. New York, McGraw Hill Medical, 2013, pp 1389–1401

Jacobson E: Depression. New York, International Universities Press, 1971

Kernberg OF: The structural interview, in Severe Personality Disorders. New Haven, CT, Yale University Press, 1984, pp 27–51

Kernberg OF: New perspectives on drive theory, in Aggression in Personality Disorders and Perversions. New Haven, CT, Yale University Press, 1992, pp 3–20

Kernberg OF: Psychoanalytic object relations theories, in Contemporary Controversies in Psychoanalytic Theory, Techniques, and Their Applications. New Haven, CT, Yale University Press, 2004, pp 26–47

Kernberg OF, Caligor E: A psychoanalytic theory of personality disorders, in Major Theories of Personality Disorder. Edited by Lenzenweger MF, Clarkin JF. New York, Guilford, 2005, pp 114–156

Klein M: Notes on some schizoid mechanisms. Int J Psychoanal 27:99–110, 1946

Oyebode F: Sim's Symptoms in the Mind: Textbook of Descriptive Psychopathology, 6th Edition. London, Elsevier, 2018, pp 83–128

Panksepp J, Biven L: The Archeology of Mind. New York, W.W. Norton, 2012, pp 95–144

Rosenfeld H: Notes on the psychopathology of confusional states in chronic schizophrenia. Int J Psychoanal 31:132–137, 1950

Searles H: Collected Papers on Schizophrenia and Related Subjects. New York, International Universities Press, 1965

Spillius EB, Milton J, Garvey P, et al: The New Dictionary of Kleinian Thought. London, Routledge, 2011, pp 466–469

Stone M: Abnormalities of Personality. New York, W.W. Norton, 1993

CHAPTER 9

Narcissistic Pathology of Love Relations

Clinical Investigation of Sexual Love and the Impact of Narcissistic Pathology

In the evaluation of patients with personality disorders, as with all psychiatric conditions, we are interested in their present-day functioning in the areas of work and profession, sexual life and love, and social life and family relations, as well as their creativity and pursuit of non-work interests. One of the most neglected of these domains is a person's sexual life. Although it is understandable that other areas may be more urgent to evaluate initially in the case of patients with a psychotic illness or an organic brain syndrome, the absence of an exploration of patients' sexual life and love relations is particularly prevalent in those with personality disorder. This is also true for a broad spectrum of patients seeking consultation because of anxiety syndromes or various types of non-major depression. Recently, there has been increased interest in one of the key components of sexual love—namely, the nature of conflictual gender identity and the general subject of gender dysphoria—but the heightened diagnostic interest in this area contrasts sharply with the lack of attention to the nature of the relationships in which patients engage for the expression of their love and sexual desire (Carroll and Mizock 2017; Yarbrough 2018). The pioneering work of Masters and Johnson (1966; Kolodny et al. 1979) showed the enormous influence that psychological—and psychologically conflictual—relationships between members of a couple has on the intensity and gratification of sexual desire. Particularly, the phases of sexual arousal, excitement, and orgasm (in contrast to the first phase of sexual desire) are powerfully influenced by the nature of the emotional relationship and the mutual interest in the love relationship of the partners. This, an almost trivial finding or, rather, confirmation of the influence that the relationship between the partners has on their sexual activity and gratification illustrates the integration of erotic desire, sexual excitement, and orgasm with an experience of love, idealization, and commitment (Kernberg 1995).

In what follows, I discuss this double aspect of sexual life: love as a relationship with a cherished person with whom sexual intimacy and tenderness have been integrated and the mature aspects of such a relationship, contrasted with the typical manifestations of patients' failure or deficits in psychopathology and couple relations in those with narcissistic personality disorder. This comparison should expand the analysis of the diagnostic features of pathological narcissism.

As part of our evaluation of personality structure and pathology at the Weill Cornell Personality Disorders Institute, we usually ask patients the following questions:

- Are you, at this time, involved in an intimate sexual relationship, involved with someone else whom you love and who loves you?
- Have you ever been in love and been involved in a long-lasting love relationship?
- Can you tell me something about the most important of these relationships and, particularly, about your present love experience?

Regardless of sexual orientation or identity, if a patient has been able to sustain any relationship over a period of time, these features can be explored. Within the broad spectrum of responses, ranging from intense emotional narratives to chaotic confusion, we would expect the aspects described in the section that follows to demonstrate a patient's optimal, "ideal" involvement in a love relationship. This is not meant to present a "norm" to which individuals must adhere, or an ideal that they must achieve, but a theoretical frame that permits us to evaluate to what extent patients have been able to establish and consolidate a love relation in their emotional life. It is prognostically and therapeutically of enormous importance in all psychotherapeutic interventions dealing with a patient's intrapsychic and interpersonal conflicts (Kernberg 2018).

SALIENT ASPECTS OF LOVE RELATIONS

One characteristic of being in love is showing interest in the personality of the loved one—an ongoing interest in understanding what one's partner is feeling, interested in, thinking about, and wishing; curiosity about the partner's aspirations and goals—and wanting to accompany the partner in these interests, even if they reflect an endeavor or activity that is not of primary interest to oneself. This interest in the living experience of the other is a privileged shared space that becomes particularly relevant at times of emotional conflicts, when serious disagreements and potential incompatibilities emerge between partners' needs. Under such circumstances, being able to put oneself into the mind of the other and look at a conflict from the other side in addition to one's own provides a perspective of understanding that facilitates the resolution of conflicts. Opening up to one's partner restores the possibility of mutual communication and compromise formations and helps to reduce resentment and prevent the deepening of conflicts through mutual projective identifications.

This type of interest is in sharp contrast to an intimate relationship in which attention is centered on "What am I getting from my partner?"; "Is he or she treating me fairly or not?"; or "Are my needs being satisfied?" Such questions reflect a tendency to internally accumulate sources of frustration and resentment about the behavior of one's partner over time. This accumulation of "justified indignation" and self-righteousness expands and waits for the next opportunity to explode.

Narcissistic patients usually evince great difficulty in describing the personality of their partners: they may concentrate on salient behavioral features about which they feel critical and on obvious superficial, conventional descriptions that do not give the interviewer a truly individualized view of the partner. At times, stressing important positive aspects of the partner that translate into the patient's own importance may highlight what, at the bottom, is causing the patient's resentment. Under normal circumstances, being interested in the internal world of the other also implies patience with the other's need to withdraw at times into his or her own inner world as part of dealing with internal conflicts or issues or with the creative spinning of ideas, plans, or images of the future. The narcissistic person, however, lacks tolerance for separateness and autonomy in the partner and may experience such temporary withdrawal as an indication of indifference or neglect.

A second characteristic of the person in love is having confidence that one's partner is interested in oneself and shares one's enjoyments, successes, and happiness as well as having a close, realistic understanding and empathy with one's difficulties, confusion, failures, and disappointments. Being able to talk with a partner about feelings of insecurity and weakness, about problem areas that one cannot resolve, and about experiences, memories, and fears that would be impossible to share with anyone else reflects trust in one's partner and a belief that one can count on the partner's understanding and empathy. In fact, wanting to share all of one's own experiences with a partner—one's interests, problems, plans, day-to-day experiences, and new understandings—is the counterpart to being interested in those of the partner. It signals a mature capacity to trust and depend on an intimate partner.

To "depend" on another in the sense of using him or her for one's own needs should not be confused with the authentic capacity to depend on a valued, close other. This is a closed area for narcissistic personalities. Depending on one's partner would mean placing oneself in a position of inferiority. For these patients, it would be humiliating to reveal their weaknesses or uncertainties. Others tend to be shadowy, existing primarily as sources of affirmation and admiration.

Third, love also involves the interest and enjoyment in doing and experiencing things together, such as social activities and friends, art, music, sports, politics, and so on. It involves sharing projects that enrich the couple's daily life, living quarters, life situation, or arrangements with children. Enjoying all of this together also involves the certainty that each partner enjoys and understands the other's need to do things alone, to have personal initiatives in which the partner is not involved, and that such temporary separation of interests does not signify a decrease in the partners' mutual love and commitment. It means tolerating each other's interest in areas in which one partner does not personally wish to participate without feeling jealousy or resentment for being excluded from that aspect of the other's life and implies an internal assurance that, eventually, whatever the other has learned or experienced will come back to the couple in a mutual sharing. Love involves a deep confidence in the permanence of the relationship through times of sharing experiences together and other times of dedication, commitment, and concern with areas of independent interests. Narcissistic personalities usually show clear indifference, if not total ignorance, about their partner's areas of personal investment and interest in which they are not involved. This lack of interest protects the patient from envying the partner's capacity to enthusiastically engage in specific tasks, studies, or creative engagements.

Naturally, if both partners are involved in different work situations or professions, such a development is a potential source of enrichment for both. Even if the partners work in the same field, they will inevitably develop different perspectives and aspects of their social environment or the nature of their work, and sharing their respective experiences may be an exciting enrichment of their work life. Here, patients with narcissistic personalities struggle with envious, competitive feelings toward the partner that may transform working in the same environment into a chronic source of resentment.

A fourth and essential aspect of love and sexual life is having an ongoing sexual interest and desire in each other, shared arousal and intensity of sexual excitement, sexual play, and interaction, and fully enjoying each other's orgasm. The experience of sexual excitement involves not only one's own subjective experience but also that of the partner, the activation of unconscious identification with each other in the sexual encounter, the unconscious expression of homosexual and heterosexual aspects of internalized object relations. It is frequently assumed that sexual interest, desire, arousal, and excitement are maximal during the early stage of a sexual relationship and tend to disappear throughout time, but this does not correspond with the experience of harmonious, long-term couples. Long-term couples in love have cycles of intense activation of sexual desire alternating with cycles of relative absence of desire and sexual activity. A periodicity of interest evolves that varies from couple to couple and in relation to the partners' ages that reflects a permanent aspect of love relations throughout life unless disrupted by external causes, such as physical illness (Hunt 1974).

The most frequent expression of narcissistic pathology in the realm of sexual experience is the effect of the unconscious devaluation of partners and gradual loss of interest in the sexual aspects of the relationship. New objects of infatuation may elicit intense sexual desire and interest, only to repeat the cycle. A long-term, habitual dissociation between emotional interest and idealization of some partners while having only erotic desire and sexual excitement for others reflects an alternative pattern of behavior that is psychodynamically closer to oedipally motivated sexual inhibition. However, both patterns may overlap and require the differential diagnosis with masochistic psychopathology.

If the partner of the narcissistic patient is a sexually responsive and emotionally mature individual, intense unconscious envy may emerge in the patient, leading to a sense of competition with the partner: who is enjoying sex more? If the partner is enjoying it more, the patient would experience this as sexual exploitation. Under ordinary circumstances, in mature relationships, the nature of sexual arousal may change throughout time, as the original idealizing of the other is gradually transmuted into the cherishing of the other as a representative of their shared sexual history. Changes that occur with time and age tend to acquire a warm, personal meaning, becoming a symbolic narrative of the relationship of the couple throughout time. The body of the other, in its changes throughout time, symbolizes the history of intimacies shared, including the growing confidence in sharing each other's fantasies and wishes and searching for new ways to gratify them. All of this is missing in the love life history of narcissistic patients.

Sexual interests and a desire for sexual involvement with others may be an unavoidable consequence of the full development of one's internal sexual freedom. Unconscious conflicts that arise within the context of a couple's social life are counteracted by the joint superego functions that protect the couple and the strength of their sexual closeness and ongoing intimate experiences. The breakdown of the couple's boundaries through extramarital affairs and various types of triangular relationships typically reflect unconscious conflicts in the couple's emotional life rather than being consequences of an unexciting and routine sexual relationship. The counterpart to being tempted to break the boundaries of sexual intimacy is the development of jealousy and intense concern when the couple's exclusive intimacy is threatened. These feelings alert the partners to possible risks to their relationship by invading third parties and motivates them to adopt protective measures to reduce and eliminate such risks.

A fifth factor in love relations is the intrinsic wish to protect the boundaries of the couple and to assert its independence from outside threats combined with a related internal dimension of mutual commitment and fidelity. Experiencing the unavoidable temptations for "triangulation" and activation of jealousy and derived protective reactions in each other and respecting and reflecting on those feelings in oneself and one's partner are important aspects of the capacity for a mature love relationship. Patients with narcissistic personalities are limited in their love investment, and thus triangulations, extramarital affairs, and multiple parallel relationships are frequent expressions of the chronic conflicts in their sexual involvements. These behaviors express chronic defensive structures against the emergence of direct aggression in these patients' dominant love relations. Their limited development of mature superego functions interferes with their ability to establish a joint couple value system that protects against the invasion by third parties, and their indifference toward their partner may become evident in their remarkable lack of jealousy.

A dimension of shared values that protect the intimacy of the couple goes together with basic honesty and trust in the benign intentional attitude of the other. Well-intentioned honesty on the part of both partners provides a frame for tolerating conflicts, disagreements, or misunderstandings. This frame protects the couple from the activation and projection of excessive aggression in either partner in escalating cycles of mutual blaming that threaten their basic trust. This superego dimension, as we have seen, is faulty or missing in the personality of many narcissistic patients.

Conflicts are unavoidable, and the most important cause of chronic marital conflicts is the unconscious activation, in both of the participants, of the dominant unresolved conflicts with their respective parental couple in the past, the permanent unconscious oedipal structure of life (Dicks 1967). These unresolved conflicts are unconsciously activated in present-day mutual projective identifications and expressions of omnipotent control in the couple's interactions, with an unconscious wish to resolve now what could not be resolved before. This simultaneous unconscious activation of unresolved conflicts of the past, with the implicit intention of resolving them by replaying them in the present, may bring about a dangerous, at times malignant equilibrium between the two respective dominant unconscious constellations, determining an intensity of conflicts around mutual aggression that may overrun the positive aspect of the love relationship. Naturally, other causes of severe chronic marital conflict may be derived from the severity of the partners' respective character pathologies, but these, in the course of their development, usually also reflect unresolved infantile conflicts and trauma. Chronic marital conflicts in which one or both partners has a narcissistic personality disorder generate the most severe and resistant of such conflicts. They raise the fundamental question of whether couples therapy is truly indicated or whether long-term psychodynamic treatment or another approach, such as transference-focused psychotherapy for one or both partners or some individualized combination of these treatments, is the treatment of choice.

One intriguing aspect of a good love relationship is the idealization of one's partner to the extent that he or she reflects aspects of an ideal parental object derived from one's early infantile idealizations, tempered and modified significantly by the evolution of one's own value systems and ideal expectations of self and others. Freud (1957) suggested that the idealization of the love object implies an impoverishment of the narcissistic investment of the self while projecting one's ego ideal onto the other. We now know that the experience of living with a person who incorporates one's ideals is an enormously enriching experience under ordinary circumstances (Kernberg 1995) and only becomes a burden in the case of individuals with narcissistic personalities, for whom such a potential idealization of the other would threaten the pathological grandiose self, or in the case of patients with borderline personality organization, particularly borderline personality disorder, for whom the lack of an integrated sense of self and of the other threatens the patient and the relationship, leading to disappointments, devaluation, and serious aggressive reactions against that supposedly ideal partner.

Patients with borderline personality disorder lack the capacity to bring together contradictory aspects of the idealized other. For very regressed patients, normal identity integration does not seem a precondition for an intense love relationship, but they cannot escape a chronically chaotic and confused relationship with their love object that precludes a stable idealization of the other. In the case of some narcissistic personality disorders, the incapacity to experience the other in an integrated way may be of very little concern to the patient, who uses the other as a kind of servant and has no interest in the internal life of the significant other. As long as the partner fulfills the patient's expectations of service and everything is taken care of, the partner drops out of the patient's mind completely. In contrast, although their commitment may be strong and steady, patients with borderline personality disorder may have to be reassured continuously of their partner's love because they do not have a solid, permanent view of the partner's personality.

A consequence of the normal idealization of the other's personality, body, and mind is a natural feeling of elation over having found the ideal partner, of experiencing the gratifying love relationship as a grace, and of a related deep sense of gratitude for the partner's existence. This gratitude may express itself in the wish to please the partner with unexpected gifts or particular gestures that demonstrate or symbolize that feeling. In contrast to conventionally expected recognition or gifts at certain fixed, culturally determined dates, such spontaneous and unregulated expressions of love and gratitude are important signals of the ongoing intimate bond of the love relationship. Narcissistic patients evince very little, if any, gratitude for the love expressed to them by their partner.

A sixth dimension of a mature love relationship is the capacity for tolerating roles that are different from and, at times, sharply contrary to those habitually enacted in the relationship. Perhaps the most typical example is the development in one, usually very independent partner, of strong dependent needs under conditions of serious failure in work or other life circumstances in which the partner seeks understanding and consolation and the tolerance and gratification of this dependence is provided by the other. Extended personal illness in one partner that transforms the other into the role of caretaker requires the capacity in both partners to accept such a dependent and even helpless circumstance as well as a natural commitment and capacity to take care of the ill partner involved in such a painful, regressive situation. This development may signify a sharp reversal of roles between a usually active and dominant partner and a more passive and dependent one. When such an extended role shift is linked to seriously threatening or terminal illness of one of the partners, it becomes a final and most challenging test of the love relationship and the commitment to it. Such a development, of course, also reflects the general destiny of all couples—their happiness together coming to an end because of the death of a partner and the other's need for physical and emotional survival. As I have pointed out elsewhere (Kernberg 2012), if the surviving partner is able to live through the mourning period and tolerate this painful life experience, he or she may be better prepared for a new love relationship, if that is still an objective possibility.

The counterpart of the capacity for accepting rapid and extreme role shifts under conditions of various life circumstances is the chronic development of conflicts around power as part of a couple's relationship. In contrast to the conventional belief in the supposedly unavoidable rivalry and power struggle between the sexes, well-functioning couples are able to establish a functional distribution of tasks and responsibilities that implies fairness, respect for and confidence in task performance delegated to the other, and the security of neither exploiting nor being exploited by the other. In a mature love relationship, the couple assumes the equality of rights and responsibilities and resolves disagreements by seeking optimal compromises that gratify, as much as possible, the wishes or aspirations of both. Their objective, in a controversy, is not "who is going to be right" but "how can we arrange for maximal gratification of both of us." This may involve career choices, balancing of work and family, child rearing, and other issues.

Whereas other types of couples' conflicts (e.g., sadomasochistic, paranoid, socially invested ideological conflicts) also may generate power struggles, this is a typical and frequent development in couples involving one or both partners with a narcissistic personality disorder. The main threat of the dominance of aggression in the life of a couple usually derives from the activation in one or both of them of unresolved persecutory past relationships with parental objects. Under such circumstances, dominant projective identifications are expressed as a vicious circle of mutual projections and splitting mechanisms that rationalize a chronic adversary relationship. The expression of unremitting needs for revenge as a fundamental source of ongoing, chronic power struggles or efforts to permanently exert control over one's partner often corresponds to features of severe narcissistic pathology, particularly the syndrome of malignant narcissism (Kernberg 2018).

Given the ambivalence of all human relations, there is a risk of actions that normally express love being unconsciously "recruited" for the service of aggression that indicates deep problems in the love relationship. At times, one partner may feel so attacked by the other that sexual desire disappears for the time being and sexual relations become limited. Conflicts around aggression are unavoidable and may constitute a healthy expression of the aggressive components of normal ambivalence in all human relations. They are acted out with the underlying security that such angry encounters do not threaten the basic relationship of love and commitment. Retrospective reflection on what caused the disagreement or outburst and recognition of one's own participation in its origin may even reinforce the love relation in the context of such angry outbursts. If the mutual sexual attraction, emotional commitment and idealization, and basic trust in the love and honesty of the other remain, acute conflicts usually are workable.

By the same token, in a mature love relationship, gratifying aspects of that relationship are not used for blackmail, in which a partner threatens to withhold an aspect of the love relationship as part of a power struggle or as a revenge move during a conflict. In such cases, sexual interaction and mutual gratification are frequently withheld by one of the partners as revenge or "punishment" for the "bad behavior" of the other, reflecting the use of aspects of love for the expression of aggression. The active refusal of sex for the purpose of control or revenge represents a power struggle in the relationship that reveals problems in the capacity for mature love in one or both partners.

The capacity to recognize inappropriate or problematic behavior in oneself or a partner and to forgive such behavior is the seventh fundamental capacity of a couple in a mature love relationship. The capacity to forgive is based on a profound recognition of experiences and concern regarding one's own past or present guilt over aggression and the related confidence that the betraying partner also has the capacity to experience guilt and the urge to repair that will constitute a new base for the relationship. This capacity may be seriously challenged, particularly in the case of marital infidelity that heavily tests mutual commitment and trust. In a couple in which one partner has narcissistic personality disorder, whatever and whoever has given cause to require forgiveness will present the couple with an extremely difficult task; if narcissistic pathology was involved, only long-term, specific psychoanalytic therapy may help the couple reach a viable resolution.

Under ordinary circumstances, the sexual relations of the couple may have important bonding functions throughout life. The sexual desire and arousal of one partner should raise sexual desire and arousal in the other and generate passionate experiences. Throughout time, growing trust and confidence in the relationship and sharing each other's sexual fantasy life permits an expansion of shared sexual fantasies and enactment and provides a private world of sexual enjoyment that, in a deep sense, constitutes a "revolution by two" (Alberoni 1987) against conventional sexuality as accepted by cultural mores. It is of interest to know what happens after sexual intercourse, and whether that experience leads to further shared intimate communication or to a satisfied mutual withdrawal "in intimacy" or, in contrast, to the isolation and dissociation of the sexual encounters from all other aspects of the couple's joint life. In contrast to conventional assumptions, intense, passionate encounters are an experience that couples share throughout their lifetime (Hunt 1974; Wallerstein and Blakeslee 1995). Individuals with narcissistic personalities may discover their potential for a passionate relationship and recover their capacity for love as a result of effective treatment. This a major objective of specific treatment for pathological narcissism and is illustrated by the extended case example at the end of this chapter.

Threats to the boundaries of the couple may evolve as their relationship becomes complicated by the arrival of children and the emergence of intergenerational conflicts, both with their respective families of origin and within their own family relationship. Here evolves the need of the couple to protect its own boundaries, its relationship against the "invasion" from these outside sources, including the demands and invasiveness that are part of normal child development. Symbolically, every parents' bedroom should have a lock on it, and their sexual life should be protected from the "threat" of intrusive advances by the children. It may seem trivial to state this; however, one major manifestation of couples' unconscious guilt over having replaced the parental families of origin and having successfully established an ideal love relationship is the enactment of unconscious guilt through the couples' self-restriction and tolerance of boundary invasions. In this way, among many others, the couple enacts oedipal guilt through masochistic, self-defeating patterns of marital interaction. The overall function of a mature love relationship is to increase the partners' enjoyment and security of life, which represents an optimal development of the human potential for love, together with an effective and gratifying support for work and profession. This is a reasonable objective for treatment, although not always possible, as we shall see in the following exploration of the psychoanalytic treatment of narcissistic personalities.

TYPICAL PRESENTATION OF NARCISSISTIC SEXUAL PATHOLOGY

A frequent, outstanding limitation in narcissistic patients is their inability to establish a mature love relationship that integrates the capacity for sexual excitement and gratification, emotional interest and commitment, idealization of the loved person, and the development of intense experiences of passionate love within such a stable, gratifying love relationship. For some, this limitation may be a motive for psychological consultation following repeated experiences of failure in intimate relationships or breakdown in marital relations and may reflect patients' awareness of missing out on an important aspect of life. Their growing sense of loneliness over the decades is a frequent consequence of the failure to establish such a fundamental link to another human being.

For others, however, this incapacity to love may only be revealed with exploration of their pathology, without the patients having been aware of it. The development of intense sexual impulses and desires for exciting new sexual relations and the experience of changing sexual partners frequently may be perceived as a major gratifying goal in life; the excitement of sexual affairs and the involvement with several partners at the same time may protect narcissistic patients from their underlying sense of aloneness. Sexual promiscuity replaces their capacity for intimacy with repeated cycles of infatuation and disappointment. This cycle may be ego-syntonic over many years before its repetition brings about chronic disillusionment and a growing sense of emptiness.

The unconscious dynamics behind this incapacity to love usually include a profound unconscious envy of the sexual partner, and, in heterosexual relations, of the other sex. A defensive idealization of sexual excitement and erotic encounters protects these patients from awareness of the deep conflicts around aggression from many sources (Kernberg 1995). Preoedipal dynamics involving unconscious desire for and envy of a perceived exciting and teasing, erotizing mother may combine with oedipal prohibitions and conflicts regarding the identification with parental images in ways that stultify oedipal resolution. In such situations, the defensive denial of oedipal reality with the fantasy of being the admired baby of a totally dedicated mother may be expressed in the patient's relationships, in which an apparent long-term couple's survival masks the total self-centeredness and unquestioned isolated superiority of the patient.

Sexual fantasies, particularly long-standing, repetitive sexual scenarios enacted in narcissistic patients' masturbatory activities, may reveal aspects of unconscious desires that, in this highly symbolic world of daydreams, are sufficiently split off from the patient's usual behavior and self-reflectiveness to reveal the underlying narcissistic conflicts. For example, one woman fantasied that no man would be able to resist her if and when she behaved seductively. Although she depreciated most of the men who had become sexually interested in her, she could respond with sexual excitement and desire to what she considered outstanding, superior, usually famous or powerful men. Successfully establishing such relationships with men with outstanding, socially recognized attributes initially gratified this patient's sense of superiority, but over a relatively brief time her growing boredom and devaluation of these ideal persons eroded her sense of triumph over all other women and pushed her to new sexual exploits. A male patient's masturbatory fantasies involved having an enormous penis that, exhibited erect on the beach, caused the admiration and sexual submission to him of all the surrounding women, who competed with each other for access to his erect penis. In some patients, the underlying ambivalence and aggression towards apparently idealized sexual partners becomes evident in their conscious fantasy life. For example, one patient had a repeated fantasy of piercing women's breasts with arrows and thus combined the excitement with women's exposed breasts with the fantasies of destroying them.

The striking lack of interest in the personality and the emotional experience of the partner is the counterpart of the narcissistic patient's incapacity to develop an integrated representation of that partner and is reflected in the dominant ongoing judgment of the partner in terms of whether he or she gratifies the patient's needs. The partner's failure to gratify the patient's needs justifies the sense of resentment and frustration that builds up in the patient with time and may be expressed by occasional or frequent rageful attacks and eventual abandonment of the partner. The loss of any interest in the partner when the excitement of novelty in the new sexual relationship wears off exposes the patient to a repeated sense of "being stuck," bored, and empty and an even less avoidable sense of aloneness.

A major typical manifestation of narcissistic relationships is the patient's incapacity to depend on the partner in the sense of being able to rely openly and trustingly and with a feeling of being taken care of, understood, and protected and to let the partner equally depend on the patient. Efforts by the partner to depend on the patient are experienced as an unfair demand; the partner should be dedicated to gratifying the patient's needs and not expect the patient to gratify the partner's needs.

The absence of gratitude in narcissistic patients for the love they receive mirrors their lack of motivation to provide pleasure and gratification to the partner. This stems from their inability to enjoy and identify with the partner's pleasure. An ongoing marriage or long-term couple relationship under such conditions presents the narcissistic patient with a sense of imprisonment in an empty life situation. Marriage may become tolerable only through simultaneous relations with other partners, a sexual promiscuity that, paradoxically, stabilizes many marital relations by allowing patients to implicitly act out their aggressive devaluation of their partner. The development of these extramarital affairs must be differentiated from other unconscious conflicts that interfere with a gratifying partner relationship and yet go hand in hand with a persistent capacity for other relationships in depth. Typical narcissistic personalities are limited in all of their object relations.

TRANSFERENCE DEVELOPMENTS

In the psychoanalytic treatment of narcissistic patients, these core features of their love lives become evident in typical narcissistic transferences. These patients have great difficulty with developing a relationship in depth in the transference. They convey an initial impression of experiencing no emotional relation to the therapist and see their treatment as a kind of business interaction in which the therapist is paid to pay attention to them and help them feel better about themselves and be more effective in their relations with significant others. That emotional distance, particularly marked at the beginning the treatment with "thick skinned" narcissistic personalities (Kernberg 2014), typically shifts into the activation of a relationship between the patient's pathological grandiose self and the devalued, split off aspects of the frustrated, traumatized, severely conflictual infantile self against which the grandiose self is a dominant structural characterological defense (Diamond et al. 2021). This transferential relationship is played out in the patient's need to maintain a sufficient sense of superiority over the therapist to feel secure in the relationship, which then threatens it by potentially devaluing the therapist in ways that would destroy the very possibility of the treatment. Efforts by the patient to maintain a certain appreciation of the therapist—while retaining a sense of implicit superiority and control—protect the patient from experiencing a role reversal in which the therapist is perceived as presenting the pathological grandiose self who enjoys superiority over the inferior and humiliated patient. This relationship, in which patients enact the pathological grandiose self in the transference, projecting the devalued part of themselves onto the therapist and then attempting to protect that relationship from a threatening reversal, is the most frequent, long-lasting, and repetitive development in the early and middle stages of the treatment of these patients.

Gradually, the underlying conflicts around conscious and, particularly, unconscious envy emerge in the transference. Usually, narcissistic patients experience envious comparison in their work and social relations that affects them severely, is expressed in a competitiveness that may create serious difficulties in their social lives, and emerges as a major threat against which their assertion of their own greatness and superiority must be maintained. That grandiosity is acted out in a subtle or not so subtle devaluation of what the therapist attempts to contribute to these patients' self-awareness and understanding of their conflicts.

Narcissistic patients have great difficulty recognizing their profound envy of the therapist, and their defensive devaluation of him or her may take the form of consciously dismissing everything the therapist says that does not coincide with their own convictions. The acting out in the transference may take the form of intellectual competition, or rapidly incorporating what they have learned from the therapist into their own, self-generated understanding, with a sense that now they do not need the therapist anymore. Patients' intellectualized imitation of the therapist's behavior and reformulation of his or her theories may serve as a way to ensure that they learn skills that will permit them to do without the therapist. This development may be particularly difficult to manage with patients who have training in psychological, even psychoanalytic understanding and who use intellectualized versions of such understanding to compete with the therapist. At worst, this development may lead to a sterile intellectualized interchange and effectively block all efforts to introspectively explore the patient's life.

For example, one patient with psychological training asserted that he would not let himself be dependent on any woman because he would not be able to tolerate the pain over separation from her. This patient had never truly experienced any pain over separations, and thus what might have been a realistic self-awareness under other circumstances was a rationalization of his awareness of his emotional non-involvement with his sexual partners. The painful experiences of conflicts related to envy may be evident in a patient's resentful sense that his or her partner is superior because the partner has rich life interests or is more attractive within the social realm. One patient who at first was proud of having an attractive wife eventually resented her for looking particularly attractive in social gatherings and obviously capturing the interest of many men. Another patient resented the friendship that her husband had with colleagues who shared his interests in certain sports and political developments and provided an intense experience from which she felt excluded. The acting out of conflicts of envy in the transference is typically represented by development of negative therapeutic reactions; for example, after long periods in which the patient complains of not being helped, a session evolves in which there is a clear breakthrough and the patient develops an understanding of some new aspects of his emotional life, which may then be followed by reinforced complaints of the uselessness of the treatment. Patients who resent the intense love that their partners feel for them because of their own incapacity to share such intense emotions may feel similar resentment in relation to the therapist's emotional availability and authentic interest in them.

Conflicts around envy may be expressed in the transference both in fantasies of sexual seduction of the therapist and in the defensive denial of any emotion or curiosity about the therapist. Frequently, women with narcissistic personality disorder have enormous difficulty developing positive oedipal transferences with a male therapist because to be interested in him means becoming dependent and therefore inferior and potentially depreciated. It is only in the advanced stages of treatment that sexual desires and fantasy may emerge in patients who previously would have experienced any such wishes or desires towards their therapist as diminishing and humiliating. However, a sense that their therapist should become interested in them sexually may represent pleasurable transference fantasies that confirm their superiority and justify their devaluation of the therapist. In the case of narcissistic homosexual patients with a therapist of the same sex, wishes for a sexual relationship may emerge as part of their need to deny envied differences and the unknowns with which they are faced regarding the sexual life of the therapist. Under conditions of intense acting out of aggression in the transference, actual attempts to seduce the therapist may reflect these patients' desire for superiority and control. Male narcissistic patients in treatment with female therapists may develop transference fantasies of seducing her as a way of asserting their superiority and disqualifying the therapist (Diamond et al. 2021).

Gradually, narcissistic patients may become aware that their rejection or dismantling of what they get from the therapist reflects their own efforts to defend against intense envy and may develop both fears of retaliation from the therapist and feelings of guilt and concern over their own aggression towards the therapist. At moments, however, the therapist also may be perceived as a good object who has not abandoned them in spite of their aggression. Paranoid transference may develop as a result, and the patients' guilt and concern about their treatment of the therapist may be expressed by intense shifts in the transference, including more open splits between idealized and devaluing experiences towards the therapist, alternations between regression into increased awareness and open expression of envy, split-off paranoid tendencies, and moments of gratitude and guilt feelings.

One patient only became aware at an advanced stage of her treatment of her tendency to resent her husband for engaging in activities that gave him pleasure instead of prioritizing whatever she wanted at that point. She realized now that this was highly destructive to their relationship and that she had assumed it was her right that he always pay attention to what she wanted, if he really loved her. She had never considered his right to do what he enjoyed even if it did not involve her. She started to feel guilty for the first time about what had, in fact, been her chronically demanding and exploitive attitude toward her husband. By the same token, she also became aware that if her husband did anything that did not fit with her wishes, she would interpret this immediately as his selfish self-concentration and attempts to control her. Another patient at this stage of the treatment became aware of the fact that his chronic irritability when getting home in the evening was linked to the fantasy that his wife and children would want him to listen to what had happened to them throughout the day, rather than considering that he had been working very hard and deserved to either be left to himself, if he so wished, or that whatever he expected for dinner or evening activities should have been taken care of rather than implying any demands on him.

Some patients develop serious depressive reactions, intense feelings of guilt, and possibly suicidal fantasies. They may begin to mourn lost or destroyed friendships and opportunities caused by their behavior. Important past relationships may emerge in this context, and patients may review long-sustained personal myths about their past that shift significantly in light of their new capacity for emotional insight. The extent to which patients are able to tolerate feelings of guilt and concern over their present reactions and behaviors both in the transference and in external relationships varies significantly from case to case. For example, one patient who held onto the image of an aggressive, controlling, cantankerous father who terrorized the family began to remember experiences of very good relations with his father and early admiration and intense feelings of love for him. These feelings had been submerged by the patient's rigidly maintained devaluation of his father's image and his unconscious identification with the negative qualities of his father as sources of power and superiority as part of his own pathological grandiose self. Another patient became aware of intense competition with his siblings that he had overcome by generally disqualifying his childhood and the social background of his family. Reflections about the past that were geared toward clarifying and confronting the long-held belief systems that were part of his pathological grandiose self evolved into a new, complex awareness of how he had repeated this past denigration and isolation from his family in relationships with his friends and his therapist.

The availability, in the patient's memory, of a good relationship that survived the overall negative and destructive scenarios of the patient's past world may become a significant positive prognostic feature. Differentiating the oedipal features of their past relationship with their parents, working through their corresponding unconscious guilt, and making efforts to repair the damaged relationship with their partner indicate patients' increased tolerance for self-reflectiveness and their efforts to free themselves from the dominance of their pathological grandiose self. Patients now may become aware and self-reflective over their past devaluation of what they received from the therapist and evince a beginning capacity to tolerate feelings of gratitude for it, and for what they receive from others, and to tolerate what is admirable in others without having to put them down. It is both a painful and a gratifying experience when patients, after years of mostly destructive and devaluing relationships, are able to discover new valuable aspects of their partner's personality that they had systematically ignored and to feel loss and mourning over good potential relationships they destroyed in the past. Patients now may become aware that they had been offered love and friendship and were unable to acknowledge, accept, and reciprocate with gratitude. The beginning of a capacity for a mature love relationship may thus emerge.

On the other hand, some patients have enormous difficulty tolerating feelings of guilt and remorse over their lack of response to love they received and their chronic mistreatment of partners. They may strongly resist relinquishing the protection provided by their sense of superiority, their fantasied capacity to take care of their own needs without needing to depend emotionally on anyone else. Some narcissistic patients are able, after many months—and sometimes years—of treatment to recognize the exploitive and sadistic aspects of their treatment of partners, but without developing feelings of guilt or concern over this behavior. To the contrary, the therapist's condescending attitude and tolerance of their behavior, with no retaliation, provides a secondary gain of defying the therapist's obvious value system and demonstrating a negative therapeutic reaction of defiance and denying guilt over their aggression. Defending themselves effectively against the painful envy of the therapist and maintaining the therapeutic relationship as the only source of safe protection against their loneliness without having to acknowledge dangerous dependency constitutes a "secondary gain" of illness. Their ongoing dependence on the relationship with the therapist, in which (in their view) the therapist is being effectively defeated, may extend stalemated treatments for years if not resolved or ended by the therapist.

This situation constitutes a not infrequent type of the syndrome of perversity, the transformation of what is given with love and concern into a source of aggression and sadistic pleasure. Sometimes this development can be worked through, and other times it cannot. Are these nonresponsive patients incapable of feeling guilt and severely limited in their moral capacity? Do some of them have undiagnosed antisocial personality disorders? Unfortunately, we have little documented material on these cases, which are referred to mostly in confidential consultations and interchange between therapists. Sometimes the dynamics of perversity can be analyzed and worked through; they obviously involve very primitive and extreme forms of envy and hatred and correspondingly difficult work for the therapist in the countertransference.

The syndrome of perversity raises questions as to when and how to determine the prognosis in such long and difficult treatments. Are there areas in which the patient presents authentic investment in values and even in people beyond his self-centered interests? To what extent is the patient able to commit to tasks that transcend personal interests? Does the patient wish to perceive herself as a good and honest person, rather than superior and triumphant? Does the patient have a clear and growing sense of loneliness? Under *optimal* circumstances, narcissistic patients may work through their intense conflicts around envy and aggression in the transference and eventually achieve the capacity for a mature love relationship, the lack of which was a major source of the chronic sense of emptiness and meaninglessness of life that they evinced at the start of the treatment.

CASE EXAMPLE: NARCISSISTIC PATIENT WITH SEVERE SEXUAL PATHOLOGY

A 35-year-old businessman originally came for a consultation because of a severe depression following his separation and divorce from his wife. He felt that his present life situation was one of deep personal dissatisfaction and loneliness despite his thriving business and longstanding success over many years. He had been referred for treatment by his internist after not responding to several antidepressant medications, and he approached me with an attitude of urgency and a somewhat desperate search for help on the one hand and a subtle grandiosity and easy activation of derogatory devaluation of what I was saying on the other, a serious contradiction between self devaluation and an air of superiority.

The patient came from a small town in the Midwestern United States, where his father was a local businessman who was respected but emotionally isolated because of his distant and withdrawn nature. The patient had feared his father because of severe punishments the patient had received from him during early childhood, but from early adolescence onward the patient had developed a strongly devaluing attitude towards him. His mother was a dominant, self-affirmative woman who was quite prominent socially but originated from a humble social background that she attempted to overcome by spreading derogatory gossip about friends and acquaintances in her present social environment. Her fundamentalist religious background was expressed in severe prohibitions and threats regarding any sexual behavior of the patient, her only son. She had been strict and controlling but always concerned about the patient's optimal functioning, pushing him to succeed at school and defending him against criticism from school authorities and, later, from friends and social acquaintances who complained about him. She was overprotective yet emotionally unavailable to the patient. He had been a good student at school and had no difficulty graduating from a leading university. Later, following the business lines of his father's work, he had developed a different area of industrial production that made him much more successful and prominent than his father had ever been.

His childhood history revealed a combination of surface submission to his dominant mother and a secret, intense, and complex masturbatory activity that gave origin to major memories he dramatized in reflection about those memories. He had spied on the sexual behavior of his parents and his neighbors and had engaged in mutual masturbation with other boys around the ages of 8–10 that had stopped, with complete repudiation of any homosexual contact, in his late adolescence. During later adolescence, he became sexually interested in girls, and since age 13 or 14 had developed intense infatuations and frequent relationships that ended after weeks or, at most, a few months because of his critical, dominant, aggressive behavior. In his adolescence, girls had rejected him, but later in life he experienced intense disappointment in and dropped women who only weeks earlier had seemed to him to be ideal. Gradually, his sexual involvements with women began to last longer as he selected women who seemed ideal to him and, in particular, were admired by other men. His personal success and prominence in college and his postgraduate engineering studies provided him with ample opportunities for establishing sexual relationships.

After years of many brief affairs, the patient fell in love with a stunningly beautiful but shy country girl he had met during a trip to a European country. She returned his love and admired his higher education and worldliness. He brought her to America, where she rapidly learned English and started college. His friends admired her for her personal attractiveness and congratulated him, and he felt pleased with the impact she made, but their marital relationship changed as she, having completed her education and established a good business position herself, became a highly appreciated and respected person in their social life. The patient became envious and resentful, felt himself diminished, and lost interest in their sexual life. He started having affairs, suggested that they have an open marriage, and eventually convinced her to participate in group sex engagements. As they became part of a social group centered on such sexual encounters, their relationship with each other weakened. Finally, following a group party where he observed his wife engage sexually with several men simultaneously, he completely devalued her and suggested divorce. The divorce triggered an intense sense of regret, loneliness, and anxiety over his future, and he then decided to consult a psychiatrist.

The patient started the treatment with a sense of emptiness, disappointment in his relationships with women, and worry over his present relationship with a new girlfriend, with whom he was already becoming bored. He experienced a growing sense of anxiety over his incapacity to maintain a good relationship with a woman. By now, most of his friends were married, had families and children, and felt satisfied with their work and profession, while he resented the ongoing emptiness and conflicts of his interpersonal relations. Despite his financial success, he was chronically concerned about whether this success would last or if he would be overshadowed by business rivals in his field. He was also losing his temporary excitement over new relations with women. He presented a strange symptom, initially mentioned in a casual manner, that eventually turned out to be quite important: sensitivity to the contact of his undershirt or shirt with his nipples and a chronic tendency to separate whatever he was wearing from directly touching them. His tugging at his shirt eventually generated in me the fantasy that he was trying to extend the contour of his body as though he had a woman's breasts. He had consulted a dermatologist on various occasions who had not found any particular pathology, and the cream the dermatologist recommended had not been helpful.

I recommended psychoanalysis, and he started that treatment with me. Rapidly emerging doubts about the efficacy of psychoanalytic treatment and questions as to what extent that treatment might help with his dissatisfaction with life, and particularly with women, gradually shifted into fantasies that, after all, his love life was probably more interesting and gratifying than that of his therapist. He envisioned me as a conventional man without any drive to compete who was rather timid in my relations with women, in contrast to his charm and certainty of success with them. He questioned my interpretive comments and reconstructed the general trend of my observations about him, triumphantly telling me that he knew ahead of time what I was going to say. In short, he developed a gradual increase of competition with me regarding the value of our "intellectual interchange" and an attitude of superiority on his part that, at the same time, created anxious feelings in him about the value of continuing in the treatment. In this connection, new information about his childhood emerged. He compared my inadequacy with that of his unavailable, distant, and uninterested father, while an identification with his mother emerged as becoming more and more dominant in his thinking, in his way of looking at the world, and in his overall derogatory attitude toward other members of his social environment. He had resented mother's powerful control and lack of emotional availability to him, and yet his sharp criticism of her alternated with admiration of her exercise of power and superiority.

In the course of the treatment, the patient established a new relationship with a woman engaged in creative art whose paintings and sculptures had raised significant interest and who also enjoyed playing the piano, an early interest that she had not pursued in recent years. As with all his other women, she was very attractive and raised attention to herself wherever she went. He was initially proud of his new girlfriend and decided that he would marry her. At the same time, faced with my questions as to whether he was repeating a pattern and to what extent he was certain of his commitment, he insisted that he was able to reach that conclusion by himself and that it had no relationship to his treatment. He now had acquired a better understanding of himself than what I was providing him.

In the middle of this development, however, profound fantasies of identification with a powerful and dominant mother emerged in his treatment, as well as memories of warm relationships he had sustained with school friends in elementary and early high school and thoughts about relationships among boys and young men that were mutually attentive and without the problems of having to pay attention and be controlled by women in order to have sexual relations with them. At that point, memories of his father shifted to his early childhood, when he had been afraid of his father as a powerful and dangerous source of punishments requested by his mother. It now appeared that his close relationships with other boys at that time and in early adolescence reflected a search for an ideal relationship with a father figure on whom he could depend, and sexual feelings for such an admired father figure emerged in connection with the memory of his adolescent homosexual experiences.

His relationship with me now oscillated between his growing sense of fear of an aggressive incompatibility in our relationship and a search for my understanding and consolation about what he now experienced as his regrets over the waste of the talents and capacities of his life. His resentment over his constant competition with others and his hatred and envy of the women with whom he had been involved earlier in his life emerged in the form of aggressive masturbatory fantasies. The nipple sensitivity, which had improved in the early stages of the treatment without our exploring it, reemerged as an important symptom, along with his awareness that what he most hated about women was their having exciting breasts and the teasing function of their exposure, being always shown and yet unavailable. He became aware of his ongoing desire to look at women's breasts, imagining how they would look naked, and he expressed fantasies that he might be able to shoot their breasts with his equipment of bows and arrows, one of his preferred sport entertainments. He felt persecuted by women as though they were in collusion to tease him. He would sit with his new wife in an open café, and women passing by on the street would attract his attention to their breasts. The combination of this interest and his resentment towards his wife because she might discover this interest in his behavior created intense anger. Masturbatory fantasies of homosexual relations in which a man would suck his penis now gave him a sense that he himself had a breast and could give milk to this man, a fantastic experience in which he could be both man and woman. Retrospectively, I believe his nipple sensitivity at this point also may have reflected a defense against the experience of an erotic homosexual transference. At that time, his envy and resentment of his business partners and relatives and, very centrally, of the remarkable talents of his new wife that he had so appreciated as something that symbolically now belonged to him, became fully available to him consciously. Paradoxically, this led to an extended period of open, vengeful devaluation of everything coming from me as a defense against such envious feelings in the transference. He had enormous difficulty recognizing his unconscious envy, which had expressed itself in typical negative therapeutic reactions, such as feeling worse after sessions in which it seemed that he had been gaining understanding of the turbulent affects that dominated his daily life.

His angry devaluation of my interpretive comments now expanded to a sense of resentment about what he felt was my indifference to him—a combination of lack of understanding and lack of concern on my part. He experienced my attitude towards him as my self-assurance, my keeping myself aloof from the problems that he had with his new wife, and when among his acquaintances in the local psychological and psychiatric profession he would tell jokes about me and my ridiculous behavior as his therapist. At first, I was not aware of this development. After several months marked by this behavior, an opportunity arose in which one of his acquaintances made an ironical observation about me that he recognized as having been formulated by him. He developed intense anxiety about this information getting back to me and preferred to "confess it" directly to me. This marked a very difficult period in the treatment, in which my intensely negative countertransference became an issue I had to resolve in the process of analyzing the meanings of his behavior. Eventually, the analysis of the transference revealed very clearly his identification with the "gossipy" aspects of his mother, one component aspect of the grandiosity and pride of his pathological grandiose self. The patient now began to experience feelings of guilt over his ongoing devaluation of me and feelings of gratitude for my not giving up on him. His reflections now included anxiety and remorse over many good relationships in the past that he had destroyed with his devaluing behavior. He also recognized, at times with a shocking emergence of feelings of guilt and concern, his devaluing attacks on his new wife.

On one occasion, as he was listening to music on the radio, he recognized the *Suite Bergamasque* by Debussy, a work that his new wife enjoyed playing quite frequently on the piano. The image of her intense concentration in that music and the profound emotional quality of love that this performance entailed overcame him, and he started to cry, both at home and again in the next session when he told me about it. A period of mourning and depression and of painful exploration of his past evolved, with a concerned and regretful attitude, deepening his awareness of his ambivalence in our relationship as well as the many ways in which he had been envious of his new wife's enjoyment of life, her creativity, and her pleasure in relations with other people. His recognition of her enjoyment and love in the relationship with him, despite all the difficulties that he was discovering in himself, gave him a deep feeling of gratitude. He started to become interested in his wife's clothing, in the many objects that she had in her space of their joint bedroom, and in what she was doing during the day. He realized how chronically inattentive of her life he had been, which signaled the beginning of a new level of their relationship.

This development marked the beginning of the completion of his psychoanalytic treatment. His nipple hypersensitivity disappeared as he became aware of his envy and resentment of women's breasts as representation of teasing aspects of very early experiences with his mother. He discovered his past wishes for closeness and permanence in the relationship with her and his always feeling rejected by her impatience with him and her apparent lack of attention to his wishes. She had conveyed the impression that as long as he did what she wanted, he could be assured that she was happy, and there was no need for any further intimacy between them. It was a world that he had recreated unconsciously in all of his relationships with women. He was now having very different interactions with his new wife, was interested in her and her life and grateful for the love that she was giving him, and shared her enjoyment with the merger of their wishes. The feelings of envy and ongoing competitiveness in his business affairs also decreased to the extent that the perennial tension at work was reduced, and he began to experience a greater pleasure in the creative aspects of his daily work. After the completion of his treatment we had no further contact until approximately 10 years later. At that time, he continued in a happy relationship with his wife, and they had one child, a son, and were satisfied with their life.

References

Alberoni F: L'Erotisme. Paris, Ramsay, 1987

Carroll L, Mizock L (eds): Clinical issues and affirmative treatment with transgender clients, in Psychiatric Clinics of North America, Vol 40–1 (The Clinics: Internal Medicine, Vol 40). Amsterdam, Elsevier, 2017

Diamond D, Yeomans FE, Stern B, Kernberg OF: Treating Pathological Narcissism with Transference Focused Psychotherapy. New York, Guilford, 2021

Dicks HV: Marital Tensions. New York, Basic Books, 1967

Freud S: On narcissism: an introduction, in The Standard Edition of the Complete Psychological Works of Sigmund Freud. London, Hogarth, 1957, pp 69–102

Hunt M: Sexual Behavior in the 1970s. New York, Dell, 1974

Kernberg OF: Love Relations: Normality and Pathology. New Haven, CT, Yale University Press, 1995

Kernberg OF: The sexual couple, in The Inseparable Nature of Love and Aggression: Clinical and Theoretical Perspectives. Washington, DC, American Psychiatric Publishing, 2012, pp 247–272

Kernberg OF: An overview of the treatment of severe narcissistic pathology. Int J Psychoanal 95(5):865–888, 2014

Kernberg OF: Erotic transference and countertransference in patients with severe personality disorders, in Treatment of Severe Personality Disorders: Resolution of Aggression and Recovery of Eroticism. Washington, DC, American Psychiatric Association Publishing, 2018, pp 215–233

Kolodny R, Masters W, Johnson V: Textbook of Sexual Medicine. Boston, MA, Little, Brown, 1979

Masters WH, Johnson VE: Human Sexual Response. Boston, MA, Little, Brown, 1966

Wallerstein JS, Blakeslee S: The Good Marriage. Boston, MA, Houghton Mifflin, 1995

Yarbrough E: Transgender Mental Health. Washington, DC, American Psychiatric Association Publishing, 2018

PART IV

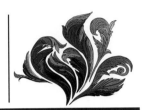

Application of Object Relations Theory

CHAPTER 10

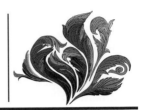

Psychoanalytic Approaches to Inpatient Treatment of Personality Disorders

A NEGLECTED DIMENSION

The contemporary psychoanalytic approaches that make use of the social experience of patients with severe personality disorders hospitalized in psychiatric specialty services started in the 1920s, with the efforts of the first generation of psychoanalytic psychiatrists in Germany to apply psychoanalytic treatment to the hospital experience of these patients. The early efforts concentrated on the utilization of patients' daily experiences to learn how to adjust to reality, carrying out concrete tasks in the

The first part of this chapter is a translation of my prologue to the text by Dulz B, Loohmer M, Kernberg OF, et al.: *Borderline-Persönlichkeitsstörung: Ubertragungs-Fokussierte Psychotherapie*. Göttingen, Hofgrefe Verlag, 2021. Copyright © 2021 Hogrefe Verlag. Used with permission. The second part of the chapter, "Recent Developments," is an overview of salient contributions of this same text.

company of other patients and using their personality resources to improve their overall social functioning. It was a treatment rooted in a long-standing tradition of inpatient German psychiatry to use hospital treatment for reeducating patients, although it was modified to include the newly developed Freudian ego psychology.

This approach also developed independently in various hospitals in Great Britain and in the United States and was expressed in a more modern form in the early programs of the Menninger Clinic in Topeka, Kansas, in the 1940s and 1950s.

Efforts to treat psychotic patients with psychoanalytic psychotherapy in a hospital setting emerged in the 1950s in the work of British psychoanalysts such as Herbert Rosenfeld (1955), who carried out such treatment with patients who were brought to his office as part of their inpatient experiences. Individual psychoanalytic psychotherapy took place relatively independently from the rest of the experience of these patients as part of their hospital treatment. A parallel effort evolved in the United States at the Chestnut Lodge Clinic, under the influence of Harry Sullivan's (1953a, 1953b) cultural approach to psychoanalytic theory. He explored the influence of early pathological experiences in family interactions that regressed patients were assumed to repeat as part of their psychotic transferences. These transferences were explored psychoanalytically in individual treatment sessions as part of the overall inpatient care. It needs to be stressed that these efforts were carried out with psychotic patients, in private psychiatric hospitals characterized by inpatient treatment of many months, sometimes up to several years' duration, at a time before the development of contemporary psychopharmacological treatments that changed this scene radically during the late 1950s and early 1960s in the United States.

The treatment of severe personality disorders, which since the 1930s had begun to be considered the "borderline" cases, opened up the question of the psychoanalytic approach to inpatient treatment as a social structure to be used as part of the overall therapeutic efforts. Early psychoanalytic explorations of borderline patients in a hospital setting were carried out at the C. F. Menninger Memorial Hospital in Topeka, Kansas, and at the Boston Psychopathic Hospital, part of the Harvard teaching system in Boston, Massachusetts. The emphasis was on ego-oriented reeducative psychoanalytic approaches, with a supportive psychotherapeutic stance, trying to achieve a more adaptive compromise between the defensive operations and instinctual impulses of these patients.

This situation changed radically with two parallel, mutually independent but eventually related approaches. One of them was the study of the hospital as a social system and the effects of a specific inpatient service culture that affected the patient and staff population. This sociological approach to the analysis of the hospital as a social system culminated in the classical work of Stanton and Schwartz (1954) carried out at the Yale Psychiatric Hospital in New Haven, Connecticut. At the same time, in Great Britain, at the Castle Hospital in London under the leadership of Thomas Main (1946, 1957), the new psychoanalytic concepts of British psychoanalysis, particularly Fairbairn's (1952) and Melanie Klein's (1946) orientations, were applied to study the vicissitudes of borderline patients, particularly the so-called special cases.

In studying the influence of the social environment of the hospital on the treatment of patients, Stanton and Schwartz (1954) found that latent, very often active but not verbalized tensions involving the medical staff, nursing staff, administrative staff, and patients' group would lead to conflicts around the management of individual patients and have a disorganizing reaction on the part of patients, particularly the special cases, as has been described by Thomas Main (1946, 1957). The idealized, persecutory, and contradictory reactions to various members of the staff and to other patients were exacerbated by the tensions generated around the care. The hidden conflicts affecting the social system of the hospital influenced the development of disagreements and conflicts regarding the management of patients with borderline conditions. Patients as individuals and as members of the particular patient culture that developed on the wards reacted in specific ways that fed into those conflicts that the staff had been unconsciously expressing in the patients' management. In short, conflicts in the social system triggered the activation of contradictory behaviors, particularly severe splitting mechanisms and projective trends among the patients. The opportunities for clarifying tensions involving the unit's entire patient group and those related to implicit conflicts among the treating staff made it possible to ventilate and resolve these conflicts, and, as a consequence, the behavior of patients on the unit showed improvement.

This work dovetailed with the discoveries at the Castle Hospital. Thomas Main (1957) described how patients with severe psychopathology, who tended to express their primitive defensive operations and interactions within the social environment, "exported" their intrapsychic conflicts into the immediate hospital environment. Splits developed among the nursing staff: a typical division of nursing staff evolved between those who had positive reactions to and were idealized by the patient and other staff members who the patient perceived in a distrustful, adversarial, and paranoid fashion and who reacted likewise, with the consequence of divisions and struggles among the staff that originated from the intrapsychic conflicts expressed in such split interactions and projections on the part of patients.

These observations evolved in the context of the newly developing knowledge of the nature of early intrapsychic developments as described by the school of Melanie Klein (1946). The fact was that, under the dominance of severe conflicts around aggression, paranoid-schizoid features of the personality were expressed in primitive defensive operations, particularly projective identification, splitting, denial, primitive idealization, and omnipotent control that now could be observed in the interactions of patients under conditions of long-term hospitalization in specialized services geared to analyze, from a psychoanalytic viewpoint, the patient's interpersonal reactions in the hospital. Rather than focusing on normalizing patients' behavior or reducing inappropriate behaviors and helping them to adjust and make use of the opportunities of work and new learning on the unit, interpretation of primitive defensive operations and object relations became the focus of inpatient treatment.

One further contribution that facilitated the analysis of these interactions between individual behavior and interpersonal development in the social field was the development of the concept of the therapeutic community, contributed to both by Maxwell Jones (1953) and Main (1946) himself. The concept of the therapeutic community emphasized the therapeutic potential of joint exploration by staff and patients, as an organized community, of all the interactions in the hospital that affected that community in total. Maxwell Jones stressed that the analysis of all activities and interactions in the community should be used in the service of the goal of reeducating and socially rehabilitating patients, providing them with new models of interpersonal interaction. Both Jones and Main stressed that living-learning-confrontation models may be used to open the flow of communication between patients and staff and to provide immediate feedback regarding observed patients' problematic behaviors and reactions.

The therapeutic community principles were expressed in small and large community meetings that, in addition, used the new information stemming from Bion's (1961) studies of group processes; his description of the basic assumptions groups of fight/flight, dependency, and pairing; and the contrast between working groups and basic assumption groups. Maxwell Jones's (1953) therapeutic community model also implied an ideal of democratic, joint decision making by staff and patients in the therapeutic community that ran counter to the traditional hierarchical model of medical treatment, a source of conflict in the application of the model. Its main orientation was sociopolitical and focused on patients learning to rearrange their social environment. Main's approach, in contrast, was heavily influenced by Bion's contribution to group psychology in which the therapeutic focus of the staff's work was the psychodynamic understanding of the patient's internal conflicts and the expression of these conflicts in split-off interpersonal behaviors on the unit that the therapeutic staff had to gather, integrate, and communicate to patients both in individual and group therapeutic encounters.

Studies by the Tavistock Clinic in London of group processes from a psychoanalytic viewpoint, and the specific development there of psychoanalytic group psychotherapy approaches based on the work of Bion, Ezriel and Sutherland, and Foulkes and Anthony, provided additional instruments for the study of group and social processes in the hospital. The Tavistock Clinic's program of Group Relations Conferences represented an important move in the direction of the application of psychoanalytic principles not only to the study of small and large groups but also to social organizations and to the psychology of organizational leadership. This work, spearheaded by Kenneth Rice (1963, 1965, 1969) and his coworkers, and its developments in the United States by Margaret Rioch (1970a, 1970b), provided an additional, crucial element in the application of psychoanalytic principles to the treatment of patients within hospital settings. All of these studies linked a functional structure of hospital organization with the setting up of specific inpatient services for treating patients with severe personality disorders.

It was the combination of all of these in the application of psychoanalytic concepts to the study of severe personality disorders—their functioning and treatment in group processes, and the interaction between the influence of intrapsychic dynamics on group processes on the one hand and of institutional dynamics on the treatment of individual patients on the other—that stimulated me to develop an integrated model of hospital treatment for severe personality disorders. I was able to develop such an approach as director of the C.F. Menninger Memorial Hospital between 1969 and 1973. This approach was continued after my departure from Topeka by Dr. Peter Hartocollis, who followed me as director of the C.F. Menninger Hospital at that point.

I was appointed medical director of the C.F. Menninger Memorial Hospital in July 1969 and was able, with the help of a distinguished group of psychoanalysts and senior colleagues, particularly Drs. Ernst and Gertrude Ticho; Drs. Lawrence Kennedy, Peter Novotnik, Peter Hartocollis; Drs. Ann and Steve Applebaum; Dr. Leonard Horwitz; and Dr. Paulina Kernberg, to develop a hospital-wide set of services geared to treat severe personality disorders. We employed a psychoanalytic object relations theory-based model that used the analytic approaches to group and organizational functioning that had been developed by Tom Main and the Tavistock Clinic under the leadership of Dr. Jack Sutherland (1952), who became a major consultant to this enterprise. We obtained the concerned, consistent, and effective support of the president of the Menninger Foundation, Dr. Roy Menninger. Because the experiences obtained in those years as part of this major experiment have been an influential contribution to the conceptual basis of contemporary approaches to the inpatient treatment of patients with severe personality disorders, I shall briefly outline the correspondent methodology.

What follows are the principal conditions and operations of this model. The patient who enters the psychiatric hospital resides in a unit that usually includes 12–25 patients, ideally not more than 30. Within the facilities of the unit, each patient needs to have a private space, small though it may be, for which he is responsible and that provides a place for his belongings that is protected from intrusions. The exception is that everything has to remain potentially open for inspections geared to avoid instruments of self-injury, danger to self or others, or that present a suicidal potential. The staff of the unit includes nursing, under the leadership of a director of nursing, and a complement of psychologists, psychiatrists, psychiatric social workers, and therapeutic activities therapists. Each patient has a psychotherapist who provides individual psychotherapy sessions, and the unit includes one to three administrative psychiatrists in charge of organizing the daily life of each patient on the unit. In teaching hospitals, psychiatric residents usually constitute part of the psychiatry staff.

The patient's day is regulated by joint activities with other patients engaged in crafts and individual creative pursuits under the guidance of therapeutic activities therapists. Each discipline has specific roles on the unit as well as a nonspecific commonly joined function. The commonly shared role implies interacting freely with patients by participating in joint activities or in the specific role relating to their profession while experiencing, in the interaction with specific patients, the impact of the patient's personality—particular countertransference reactions that emerge in the ongoing context and interactions on the unit. There are staff meetings dedicated to sharing the impressions that patients make on staff and the countertransference reactions that are generated in the contacts with patients. In these meetings, very different impressions and reactions to patients may be shared, and the predominant primitive mechanisms that patients with severe personality disorder evince may become clearly evident.

The effects of patients' projective identifications—splitting staff into idealized and persecutory objects and the aggressive, derogatory behavior of patients, as well as their timid or desperate search for support and company, conflictual dependency needs as well as efforts to omnipotently control the environment—may become evident in the mutual sharing of experiences of the staff.

Patients meet not only in task groups that carry out the work functions that permit staff to observe patients' interactions and overall capacity to function within a social group but also in daily living group meetings in which problems that have emerged in living together on the unit can be discussed, particularly difficulties and conflicts that have emerged involving patients and staff, and can be examined from multiple perspectives. Once a week, a general community meeting of all patients is joined by the entire staff and focuses on issues that affect the entire patient–staff community of the unit. The full participation of patients and staff permits an immediate sharing of all information broadly and clearly.

The patient's psychotherapists may be members of the same staff or come from outside the unit. In either case, it is important that a mechanism exists that informs the therapist of all the interactions of his patient in between the individual sessions, so that the patient's life during the entire day, day by day, on the unit may be available for exploration and analysis of the reactivation of his problems in the context of the unit.

The exploration of primitive conflicts and defensive mechanisms occurs in the "here and now." Although elements of the patient's past may be important to be known by staff and, particularly, the therapist and to be included, when relevant, in the analysis of the activation of present problems on the unit, the task is to help patients to understand their present experiences, behavior, interactions, and suffering, as well as their potential and difficulties, and thus prepare them for continuing this psychotherapeutic venture after leaving the hospital.

An important variation of this model may be the use of psychoanalytic group psychotherapy that, in contrast to exploring the day-to-day living problems on the unit, would be conducted strictly according to a technical approach developed on the basis of some degree of modification of Bion's model of group analysis. This is not the place to discuss technical details that differentiate the Bionian approach (Bion 1961) from the Ezriel-Sutherland approach (Ezriel 1950; Sutherland 1952), or Anthony and Foulkes's approach (Foulkes and Anthony 1957). Whichever of these techniques is utilized, it is important that the consistency of the technical approach of the group psychotherapy has a clear relationship to the individual psychotherapy of patients, that the risk of an excessive dilution or splitting of transference developments be avoided, and that the integrative function of the individual psychotherapy be preserved. It may happen that the intensity of frequent psychoanalytic group psychotherapy sessions practically replaces the individual psychotherapy, but that is an open question. In any case, the fact that each patient has a psychiatrist with an administrative function regarding the total development of the treatment on the unit should protect the treatment from fragmentation and inconsistencies.

An important aspect of this treatment approach is the relative freedom of staff to interact with patients, both in their specific roles and in their nonspecific human availability. That requires specific training, a certain degree of maturity, and, above all, an internal sense of freedom on the part of staff to share their reactions to patients with each other so that these reactions may be used to explore the total expression of the patients' intrapsychic experiences activated in the interpersonal interactions during the hospital stay, by means of transference and countertransference analysis.

One important precondition for the development of such a program is a commonality of understanding patients' psychopathology, of the nature of the exploration of this pathology on the unit, and of the nature of the therapeutic approach to patients, all of which requires not only training, knowledge, and experience but also a facilitating hospital environment.

It is indispensable that a respectful, functional, nonauthoritarian atmosphere prevail in the unit's functioning, in contrast to an authoritarian, paranoiagenic atmosphere of intense fear, ambivalence, and resentment towards authority within the staff that would militate against the possibility of open communication among staff in reaction to patients' development. Such a functional, nonauthoritarian atmosphere requires functional leadership on the part of the unit director, usually a psychiatrist, and a collegial relationship between the members of the team that transcends their individual professions. A truly interdisciplinary working team enriches the specific functions of each of the staff members. The development of such a functional atmosphere, in turn, requires a support of this program on the part of the hospital leadership beyond each unit, an atmosphere of collegiality between the various units or services, and a functional hospital administration that includes a participatory management style in which struggle around resources, time distribution, delegation of authority, and administrative control can be openly and functionally negotiated and resolved.

The experience at the Menninger Hospital in which this program was developed indicated the definite possibility of installing such a treatment program. I had the support as medical director of the hospital (my role during the 4 years in which I developed that program) and the support of the overall leadership by the president of the Menninger Foundation and his administrative department. To set up such a program as an isolated empirical trial in the context of an adversarial hospital administration would condemn it to failure. In fact, the effort to reproduce this model in various other places indicated that one of the risks of such a program is the development of an "ideal working environment" within an island of innovation that inspires an institutional envy and jealousy, resentment, and ambivalence throughout the rest of the institution not involved in the program that tends to undermine it. It also needs to be stressed that the arrangements described imply a degree of functional leadership but not a politically "democratic" system. In this regard, the program differs markedly from the therapeutic community model proposed by Maxwell Jones (1953) and is compatible with a "traditional medical model" as long as that does not reflect a euphemism masking the authoritarian distortion of a contemporary, functional medical model.

Another important risk for such a program is the very gratification of working in an open, humanly respectful and interested environment that tends to bring staff close to each other and fosters a potential increase in the aspiration for gratification at work for which a price may have to be paid. In fact, excessive idealization and commitment to such an "ideal world" may lead to significant activation of complex interpersonal expectations and conflicts among staff and, eventually, to the typical "burnout" syndrome that results from an excessive idealization and work commitment that replaces ordinary living outside of the work situation for some or many members of the staff.

The 1960s and 1970s may be considered the high point of the development of "milieu" programs in the United States similar to the one described, as new knowledge regarding psychoanalytic object relations theory, group processes, and organizational management, and the utilization of the social environment for therapeutic processes was integrated into inpatient programs. Potential constraints of these programs pointed to their limitations. These include, first, the need for a highly sophisticated and trained staff, which is not easy to reproduce in many parts of the world; second, the relatively high staff investment in this program, which is complicated by the intense amount of time required by various group meetings, further stressing the available staff time in spite of high staffing; third, the conditions required regarding the environmental surroundings of such specialized programs, the facilitating atmosphere at the level of the broader institution in private as well as state or federal psychiatric facilities.

At the same time, several realities developed that curtailed these programs, perhaps with a particular impact in the United States. First, the development of psychopharmacological treatment, which was mostly helpful with psychotic illness, particularly schizophrenia and major affective disorders, reduced interest in the psychoanalytic psychotherapy of psychosis within psychiatric hospital settings. The initial expectations that similar positive psychopharmacological results might be achieved with severe personality disorders brought about a problematic overemphasis on the psychopharmacological treatments of these latter conditions and raised questions about the usefulness of their intensive, long-term inpatient treatment. Third, and most importantly, the development of the community-based psychiatry movement in the 1970s and 1980s led to shorter inpatient stays and a shift of public and private reimbursement dollars to outpatient (less costly) treatment. Ironically, psychotic patients were being discharged with the help of psychopharmacological treatment but without the availability of the promised community resources, resulting in a significant chronic psychotic patient population living in bad psychosocial circumstances within communities. The reduction of hospital beds and hospital staffing naturally affected services geared to the long-term treatment of severe personality disorders as well. The advent of "managed care" in the United States was a major force that, driven by economic necessities, tended to dramatically reduce the length of stay of inpatient treatment and brought about its assumed replacement by mostly psychopharmacological outpatient treatment for the population of severe personality disorders as well, with the disappearance over the 1990s of practically all long-term inpatient services for severe personality disorders.

The development of cognitive behavior–oriented treatments for severe personality disorder constituted another important element of the changing scene in the 1980s and 1990s. The effectiveness of dialectic behavior therapy (Linehan 1993) in the treatment of suicidal and parasuicidal symptomatology of borderline patients cemented its economic viability and effectiveness by the fact that the corresponding techniques could be learned in a brief period of time by a broad spectrum of staff, and treatment duration could be reduced. The development of group psychotherapeutic methods that provided an alternative for financially viable long-term outpatient treatment for severe personality disorders was undermined by insurance companies' concern that the cost of long-term individual psychotherapy might be replaced by that of long-term group psychotherapy as well! Increased bureaucratic requirements regarding the conditions and documentation for long-term group psychotherapy managed to practically eliminate this modality of treatment, other than within the time restricted limits provided by brief cognitive-behavioral approaches.

One brilliant exception to this general trend is provided by the residential treatment setting of the Austen Riggs Psychiatric Clinic in Stockbridge, Massachusetts (Plakun 2011). This clinic has developed a sophisticated, psychoanalytically oriented long-term treatment program that combines individual psychoanalytic psychotherapy with an analytically oriented therapeutic community program geared to the treatment of severe personality disorders, creatively using the various psychoanalytic group modalities referred to above.

It is in the context of this culturally negative environment that the development of the treatment of severe personality disorders, both regarding individual psychotherapy and hospital management, survived under the influence of a few highly specialized research efforts that proved to be successful.

Moving from Topeka, Kansas, to the Department of Psychiatry of Columbia University in New York in 1973, I developed an inpatient program at the New York State Psychiatric Institute based on the model that had been carried out at the Menninger Foundation. Over several years, a group began to consolidate, including Dr. Michael Stone, Dr. Steven Bauer, Dr. Howard Hunt, Dr. Catherine Haran, and myself, that focused on developing the conceptualization of borderline personality organization—that is, the common psychopathological frame of severe personality disorders—and on developing an updated psychoanalytically based psychotherapeutic approach to these conditions, with particular application to inpatient settings. We also focused on training psychodynamic psychotherapists, given the fact that all psychiatric residents at the Psychiatric Institute rotated for the entire third year of training in that service.

In 1976, following an invitation from Dr. Robert Michels, chairman of the Department of Psychiatry of the Weill Cornell Medical College, to become the medical director of the Westchester Division of the New York Hospital and to develop the programs that I had originally developed at the Menninger Hospital, our entire group, including Dr. Arthur Carr, originally director of psychology at the Psychiatric Institute, Dr. Michael

Stone, Dr. Steven Bauer, Dr. Catherine Haran, and myself, moved to the Westchester Division and set up an inpatient service with the characteristics of the specific psychodynamic inpatient service for severe personality disorders referred to before (Kernberg 1998, 2012). In the course of the next few years, we were joined by Dr. John Clarkin, with his particular expertise in research design, who became principal investigator of our empirical research projects. Dr. Frank Yeomans became the director of the specialized inpatient service for borderline personality organization at the Westchester Division, and Dr. Catherine Haran joined him as director of nursing at that service. Over the next 20 years, we continued our learning and understanding of personality disorders and their treatment. In 1996, upon my retirement as medical director of the hospital, the Personality Disorders Institute (PDI) at the Westchester Division was created by Dr. Jack Barchas, the new chairman of the Cornell Department of Psychiatry. The creation of the PDI, under the auspices of the Department of Psychiatry, allowed our group to continue our psychotherapy and empirical research.

The PDI developed research projects studying the psychopathology of borderline personality organization, new methods for the clinical evaluation of patients, and, eventually, the development of transference-focused psychotherapy (TFP), a specific psychoanalytic psychotherapy geared to the treatment of patients on the borderline spectrum (Yeomans et al. 2015). Several randomized, controlled trials clinically confirmed the effectiveness of TFP and represented a significant contribution to the psychodynamic treatment of these highly prevalent, severe psychopathological conditions. Furthermore, we developed an updated systematic psychoanalytic group psychotherapy approach applying TFP in a group setting that, in essence, represented some updated modification of the Ezriel-Sutherland approach (Kernberg 2012).

Given the mounting pressures to reduce length of hospital stay, the requirements of managed care, the reduction of personnel in inpatient services, and the development of cognitive-behavioral models for group treatment geared to short-term hospital stay, our psychodynamic program shifted to the outpatient treatment of severe personality disorders. It remained a task for countries in which the much-needed extended inpatient treatment for severe personality disorder could be continued to develop further corresponding psychodynamic treatment programs. It has become clear, in the meantime, that the treatment of severe personality disorders is essentially psychotherapeutic and that medication has only an auxiliary therapeutic function and cannot replace the need for intensive, specialized psychotherapeutic treatment. Ironically, the systemic move away from lengthy inpatient stays has brought about the phenomenon of frequent, repetitive hospitalizations for these patients. It is not uncommon to see patients who have had 10, 20, or more inpatient hospitalizations along with frequent use of emergency services.

These repetitive, discontinuous, brief inpatient treatment episodes usually undermine any constructive approach that would attempt to consolidate the patient's capacity to function in the world, including an ongoing long-term psychotherapy with the same therapist. The need for extended-care inpatient programs for severe personality disorders has clearly become evident, but its implementation, at this time, is seriously limited in many parts of the world, including the United States. The opportunities for the development, updating, and improvement for these treatments resides presently in European psychiatric hospital settings.

Space does not permit my articulating the essential characteristics of TFP, but permit me to refer you to our manual, *Transference Focused Psychotherapy for Borderline Personality Disorder* (Yeomans et al. 2015).

What follows is a brief summary of the group psychotherapeutic frame derived from TFP that may constitute an important component of both inpatient and outpatient treatment for severe personality disorders.

Group TFP is based on the approach of Ezriel and Sutherland (Ezriel 1950; Sutherland 1952) and a modification of Bion's (1961) original approach to group analysis. Ezriel and Sutherland combined the analysis of predominant group themes and the analysis of the position individual patients adopt regarding the conflicts activated in the corresponding basic assumptions groups. The overall technique, in short, involves the group leader inviting patients in the group to talk freely about "what comes to mind" and to observe their reactions while in the process of the psychotherapeutic group situation, with the expectation that the basic assumptions group developments will evolve in the direction of fight/flight, dependent, or pairing group orientations.

The group leader, while pointing out the nature of the basic assumptions group activated in the group setting, would point to the extent to which the contradictions in the reaction of various group members toward this group situation reflected the underlying unconscious conflict now affecting all members of the group. Following Ezriel's recommendation to signal the predominant group tension as a reflection of a "required attitude" within the group that expresses a defensive function against an opposite, "avoided" experience of the group (an avoided experience that might bring about a calamitous situation and corresponding relationships that have to be avoided), the therapist would interpret this conflictual theme. He then would go on to point out how individual members react to this common theme in terms of their individual dispositions toward the conflict. In this process, the group therapist maintains a position of technical neutrality, attempting to diagnose the dominant themes when the situation seems right for doing that and only following the general clarification of the group situation with a sequential pointing to individuals' position adopted within that general tension.

In short, the main strategy of the TFP group psychotherapeutic approach is to facilitate the interpretation of the basic assumptions group in the context of the nature of the primitive object relations and related defensive operations activated in the course of the group development. Rather than interpreting the sequential activation of individually determined dominant transference dispositions in the course of the group sessions, the therapist's interest is on the sequence of the group processes, the progressive and regressive fluctuations of group tensions that facilitate activation of particular conflicts in individual patients by means of their "valence" in the group at different times. This approach facilitates addressing individuals at a point when their individual psychopathology is particularly activated under the impact of a certain common group tension, so that the TFP principle of interpreting affectively dominant conflicts holds for both the analysis of the group tension and the analysis of the position of key members of the group in the enactment of conflictual reactions to this common group tension. The therapist's interventions in the group are guided by the same principles as the interventions in individual TFP sessions: first, by what is affectively dominating the group; second, by the nature of dominant transferences operating within the group atmosphere; and third, by his or her countertransference.

The therapist's maintenance of an attitude of technical neutrality regarding developments in the group is limited by establishing clear rules about what is not tolerated, particularly, physical aggression against the therapist, the group members, or physical property; gross sexual harassment; and self-destructive behaviors, such as self-cutting or burning. The techniques used are interpretation, transference analysis, technical neutrality, and countertransference utilization, which follows the general principles and guidelines of the technical approach of TFP. The overall strategy of highlighting and resolving the affective dominance of these patients' dissociated primitive internalized object relations is systematically employed in the order in which these object relations achieve dominance as part of the group regression.

In conclusion, there are patients with borderline personality organization whose severity of regression, lack of capacity to participate in an outpatient psychotherapeutic treatment, negative prognostic indicators (such as severe antisocial features or secondary gain of illness), and complicating symptoms such as alcoholism or addiction may require specialized long-term inpatient treatment. This, eventually, would make continuing this treatment on an outpatient basis possible, particularly as TFP is geared to change the total personality structure and not only to obtain symptomatic improvement. The methods developed in the experience of inpatient treatment of borderline patients that have been summarized here are available for further development. They promise to expand our overall effectiveness in the treatment of these conditions, in contrast to shortsighted attempts to reduce treatment time and efforts in brief inpatient hospital interventions only geared to temporary symptom reduction.

Recent Developments

Although long-term inpatient treatment in specialized settings for severe personality disorders has practically disappeared in the United States, it has continued to be a significant aspect of the treatment of these disorders in Europe, particularly in Germany, Switzerland, and The Netherlands. An important recent overview of these programs by Dulz et al. (2021) provided a description of these developments, particularly the application of a TFP model for the intensive treatment of these patients in specialized inpatient units. What follows is a brief overview of these developments as summarized in Dulz et al. (2021). The corresponding experience of the authors derives from their work in hospitals in Basel, Hamburg, Munich, and Münsterlingen. In addition to their having integrated the pioneering experiences carried out in the United States that were summarized earlier in this chapter, they refer to the as-yet limited empirical research on the effectiveness of these treatments (Agarwalla et al. 2013; Dammann et al. 2016; Häfner et al. 2001; Solberger et al. 2014). General criteria for the indication of inpatient treatment of borderline patients include the development of regressive crises in borderline patients that seriously affect their capacity to function in an outpatient setting, particularly severe suicidal risks that cannot be controlled by the usual structuralization of outpatient treatment; dangerous, life-threatening, self-destructive behavior; total breakdown of the capacity for social interactions (including their incapacity to work as well as long-standing social isolation); comorbidity with other disorders frequently linked with severe personality disorders, such as addiction and severe eating disorders; and chronic and severe negative therapeutic reactions. Inpatient treatment also may be indicated for patients with demonstrated failure to improve with a spectrum of both cognitive-behavioral and psychodynamic psychotherapies, carried out with an appropriate level of competence, in ambulatory treatment efforts.

While hospitalization for acute regressions may require only a brief inpatient stay, this is also the case with patients whose chaotic environmental situation requires temporary separation of the patient from such environment. All the other indications mentioned are indications for the long-term inpatient treatment that is explored in this European approach (Dulz et al. 2021). Patients with a combination of major depressive illness and characterologically based depression, particularly when such depressions are chronically resistant to treatment and complicated by suicidal tendencies, may require careful evaluation as to what extent brief diagnostic hospitalization should be shifted into the kind of long-term program represented by inpatient TFP.

Potential contraindications for this treatment, in addition to severe restriction of patients' cognitive capacity, would be severe delinquency and the corresponding risks for patients and staff in an inpatient setting.

The treatment setting is a specialized unit of usually 25–30 patients' capacity, with a selection of patients presenting a broad spectrum of personality disorders and excluding both acute and chronic organic mental disorders as well as long-lasting psychotic disorders other than the brief psychotic episodes that severe personality disorders may evince, particularly under the influence of comorbid substance use. The unit staff, nurses, nursing assistants, activity therapists, and educators, as well as psychologists, social workers, psychiatrists, and administrative staff related to the unit, all should obtain education in the basic principles that underlie TFP. This training should include contemporary psychoanalytic object relations theory, the psychodynamic understanding of the psychopathology of severe personality disorders, and the general principles of a psychodynamically oriented approach to patients that is attentive to transference and countertransference. The ongoing communication and elaboration of this knowledge by unit leadership is considered an essential aspect of the treatment structure of the unit, and clinical examples given by patients' pathology are continuously used to illustrate the application of these theoretical approaches in interactions with patients.

The predominance of primitive defensive operations will bring about significant splitting of staff initiated by patients' interaction. The effect of massive projective identifications in the distortions of the perception of social interactions on the unit and the complex interaction on the part of patients have to be assumed as unavoidable aspects of life on the unit. The combination of maintaining a structured social environment while tolerating the development of regressive reactions and interactions from a position of technical neutrality is a key element of the management by staff of the unit. Emotional containment of the tensions initiated by patients' interactions among each other and with staff is an important aspect of the study of the significance of these interactions and for tracing them back to individual patients' psychopathology. The general treatment objectives covering all patients include, at first, to stabilize their functioning within the routine of the daily life of the unit, and second, to assess the individual motivation and lack of motivation for treatment as a first indicator of at what level of interaction the patient can be approached and how the patient's motivation can be reinforced.

The treatment process usually lasts approximately 3 months. It is initiated by a preliminary discussion with patients and families about the diagnosis of the illness and the purpose of inpatient treatment and involves a very careful diagnostic evaluation with structural interviewing and the related diagnostic instruments. A general contract established with the patient spells out the conditions under which the patient will enter this 3-month inpatient treatment and his understanding that he will be both in individual treatment and participating in general therapeutic activities.

Treatment can be divided into three major periods: the first 2 weeks focus on adaptation to the program, followed by a middle phase of approximately 6 weeks in which the program is carried out, and a transitional and termination phase of approximately 4 weeks. During the initial period, individualized treatments are initiated, particularly in the case of suicidality, alcoholism, drug dependency, and self-mutilating activities. The individualized treatment of these complications differentiates patients' treatment and will determine the priorities of their daily activities.

The unit has a clearly defined social structure that includes a daily program of joint activities. Social rules include the expectations for dress code and presentation; shared responsibilities for cleanliness, hygiene, and order in patients' rooms and joint group rooms; the rules of interactions with other patients that limit the tolerance of aggression and assure appropriateness of sexual and intimate behavior; and visiting hours, mealtime, play time, television time, and the times reserved for rounds and group meetings. Patients are instructed not to discuss the problems of other patients outside the group meetings, to maintain confidentiality regarding all visits from outsiders, and to feel responsible not only for their own well-being but for that of the community. The clarity of the assumptions of these regulations of material life on the unit naturally enters in conflict with the acting out of the patients' internal conflicts. Corresponding issues, including tolerance of others, love and sex, respect and discretion, and politics and religion, all are sources of expression of patients' conflicts that are controlled within the social boundaries of the community while providing material for their exploration in individual psychotherapy sessions.

During the initial phase of the treatment, relatively few expectations are made for patients' individual behavior. Their program is structured individually in terms of their personal interaction with staff and their participation in group meetings. Patients' individual TFP psychotherapy is carried out by a specialist M.D., Ph.D., or M.S.W. who is a staff member of the unit, for two sessions per week. The psychotherapists participate in meetings in which their patient is centrally discussed. These meetings include a general conference about the patient's condition, development, and treatment after approximately 3 weeks on the unit. At that point, all the information that has been gathered can be communicated to the patient's psychotherapist, who, in turn, can communicate what he thinks is important and what staff should know in terms of major object relations dominance in the patient's present experience. These dominant object relationships of the patient become shared information of all the staff involved with the patient, to be worked on in the patient's interactions with staff and other patients. Major objectives are established in terms of what kind of object relation conflicts need to be explored, which are very often not those that the patient believes are his main problems. For example, patients who come with a firm conviction that all their troubles derive from sexual abuse suffered in their childhood may learn that other issues are now the central focus of their difficulties. All the members of the team treating the patient work on the particular affectively dominant object relationships that are the main present manifestation of his psychopathology.

By the mid-phase of treatment, the patient and staff should have a clear notion of the typical dyads that represent the patient's transference, and related staff countertransferences, that can be examined from a position of technical neutrality. Practically, from the viewpoint of TFP, staff should have a realistic awareness of the patient's deeper problems, and the clarification and confrontation of the patient's behavior by all members of the team and in the group therapy signal the general awareness and participation of the social system of the unit in the patient's treatment. One particular method facilitating this interaction is the "reflective team." This method refers to team discussions about and with the patient, and each patient has the opportunity for one such conference a week.

In the transitional and final phase of the treatment, issues of separation and sadness over leaving the unit and orientation to external life are taken up, often in the context of the reappearance of symptoms that had improved in the course of the inpatient treatment.

As previously mentioned, patients receive individual psychotherapy twice a week with standard TFP techniques. The therapist, as part of the treatment, explores his dual roles as therapist and as part of the administrative structure of the unit as a given of the inpatient treatment structure. The leadership of the unit provides the ultimate authority for the management of the patient. Group therapy and individual therapy are maintained completely separately, so that group therapy is clearly differentiated from the reflective team structure and from community meetings in which day-to-day problems of the unit are explored. Group therapy maintains its own structure by the specific analysis of the developments within the group itself.

The group TFP component of the program is a complex development of the psychoanalytic group therapy derived from Bion's (1961) and Ezriel's (1950) approaches. In general, the group should have two leaders who can help each other in the complex analysis of group developments implied in this approach. The group therapy has two combined ways of dealing with the activation of patients' predominant internalized object relationships. One major focus is the expression of each patient's affectively dominant internalized object relations towards other patients of the group and the active exploration of group members' mutual interactions as an expression of the interaction of their corresponding dominant internalized object relations. At the same time, group leaders also pay attention to *total* group regression, that is, the "basic assumption group" regression expressed in Bion's approach to group analysis. The analysis of the activation of basic assumption groups, combined with the analysis of predominant individual interactions among patients, characterizes the content of each group session. There is no analysis of the group's reactions to the leader nor of the individual group members to the leader, so that internalized object relationships are clearly focused on mutual interactions among patients, which is reminiscent of Ezriel's approach, combining the analysis of dominant group themes, group resistances, and "avoided subjects" with how these developments affect every patient. It is an original application of TFP that clearly differs from the earlier development of our model of group psychotherapy in the United States. The interpretation of hypothesized object relations dyads and the reaction of the individual group members to the discussion of these dyads become important means of learning that complement the individual experiences with staff throughout the rest of the day.

A community meeting of all the patients is held on a daily basis, directed by a member of the staff or by a patient. The discussion focuses on the daily life on the unit, on planning activities, exploring problems, and greeting new and departing members of the group. At the beginning and end of the week there are team meetings in which all administrative issues, shifts, and responsibilities are discussed and, again, particular problems that need to be explored are analyzed from the viewpoint of the activation of internalized object relations in patients and their interactions. Once a week a clinical meeting takes place in which a case is discussed in depth and in which team leadership provides information, teaching, and decisions that need to be made at an administrative level. These meetings assure the high standard of work on the unit. Once a week each individual patient meets with a team to discuss his development on the unit, and these meetings are confidential. No other patients can be present. This also gives patients a chance to express their general view of the unit, their satisfactions or dissatisfactions.

The overall direction of the program by the unit chief includes his responsibility for the harmonious relationship between the unit and its surrounding environment. Typical conflicts arise between the special conditions of the unit and the general philosophy and problematic interactions between unit and the "external world" of the hospital at large.

The nursing staff has multiple functions as part of this program. Nursing staff have to organize the daily life on the unit, observe patients' interactions, maintain the social structure of the unit, and provide documentation of patients' development. They have to protect viability of the "real space" of patients' informal interactions, coordinate the individually different forms of therapy that patients are engaged in, deal with crises in the social interaction of the unit, and stabilize the unit in the context of regressive developments. In addition, they have a specific function with individual patients in the sense that each patient receives the assignment of one member of the nursing staff to be available to him to discuss in a weekly meeting all the issues, program activities, and relationships with other patients that affect the patient and to permit the patient and the member of the nursing staff to clarify specific problems and how to deal with them. The assignment nurse informs the patient of how he is perceived on the unit and what kind of problems he may be facing of which he may not be aware. In these individual relationships, the staff person should react spontaneously and authentically, confronting the patient with the transferential aspects of his behavior, supporting his capacity for empathy with others, and including partial communication to the patient of the staff person's countertransference. This contributes to the reality testing of the social situation on the part of the patient and increases his capacity both for empathy and understanding. As a general rule, all staff interfacing with patients are trained to delicately reflect to the patient the effect of his behavior on others, including the staff. To the extent that the patient can make positive use of this feedback to moderate his behavior, his relations with fellow patients and staff will show improvements. Not all patients are able to tolerate this feedback, and their relations remain discordant. These are delicate, open, and remarkably free interactions that require high-level training of staff and constitute a potentially important learning experience for patients.

As mentioned before, team meetings take place in which debriefing of staff helps in the containment of countertransference reactions, an important complementation of these intense interactions with patients. It is important that staff communicate their reaction to patients not as a discharge of their own emotional needs but clearly from a position of technical neutrality, and this requires an enormous degree of tact and timing. An important part of what happens on the unit occurs, of course, at night, with fewer staff available and more opportunities for acting out by patients. Night incidents have to be considered seriously and explored in the group interactions in which the daily life of the unit is discussed.

The role of the social worker is the establishment and elaboration of the contact between the life on the unit and the patient's maintained relation with external reality. The psychiatric social worker has an important role in observing the extent to which external reality continues influencing the patient. The patient's reality represented by his family, work situation, and intimate relationships has been disrupted by the inpatient treatment, and enriching the awareness of external reality sharpens the therapeutic focus for patient and staff. This prevents the patient from remaining aloof from the therapeutic milieu by focusing only on his external life or cocooning into a complacent identity as a "mental patient," happy to live in such a protective environment.

Specific individualized therapies that patients may engage in, in terms of their particular pathology, capabilities, interests, and talents, include social relations and organization of activities with other patients, development of individual creative talents while on the unit, participating in specific work therapy, physical therapy, art therapy, and development of specific products. The patient's behavior is explored in terms of collaboration, activities, effectiveness, and his creative work. In this context, skills training and psychoeducation may be included and can be combined with a psychoanalytic approach that stresses the importance of the exploration of internalized object relations. Nursing staff has to be trained to be able to provide skills training and psychoeducation for helping the patient in his daily life but without attempting to reduce, by cognitive-behavioral methods, the patient's anxiety and conflicts with significant others that reflect the activated internalized object relationships. Specific training, work, and social activities permit a supportive approach that is clearly differentiated from the constant attention to intrapsychic issues involved in the patient's interpersonal tensions and conflicts on the unit.

An important aspect of the general maintenance of the social structure of the unit is the restraint of staff in reacting with excessive rigidity and strictness to correct "bad behavior" or pressing towards discharge of patients who have created intense negative reactions. On the other extreme, there is a risk of excessive flexibility when trying to provide tolerant understanding under conditions in which the patient's severe regression threatens the maintenance of the social structure of the unit. Ongoing internal supervision by the leadership of the unit and supervision of individual patients, including inviting external consultants if necessary for extremely difficult cases, maintaining an appropriate combination of firmness, and maintaining the social structure without giving in to extreme countertransference reactions, is part of the task. Problems that create these alternative reactions include sexual relationships between patients and the need to evaluate to what extent intimate relations between patients may be therapeutically workable and therefore can be tolerated or the extent to which the dangerous exploitation of patients by others requires discharge of a particular patient. Delinquent actions on the unit, such as patients who steal from others, equally may be explored in terms of whether the antisocial behavior is workable or threatens the unit to an extent that the patient needs to be discharged. It is important to protect team members from threatening patients, and it has been generally found that antisocial personality disorders in a strict sense have a counterindication for this treatment approach (as probably for all psychotherapeutic treatment approaches). Patients whose extreme passivity and "pseudostupidity" signify an unchangeable waste of their time on the unit may occasionally also lead to an early discharge. The interplay between technical neutrality, active interventions to protect the social structure, confrontation of the patient's acting out, therapeutic management, and respecting the limits of the capacity of containment in specific situations are challenging tasks for the staff, and the motivation for further development of this therapeutic method.

References

Agarwalla PA, Küchenhoff J, Sollberger D, et al: Ist die stationäre störungsspezifische behandlung von borderline-patienten einer herkömmlichen psychiatrischen/psychotherapeutischen stationären behandlung überlegen? Schw Archiv Neurologie Psychiatrie 164(6):194–205, 2013

Bion WR: Experiences in Groups. New York, Basic Books, 1961

Dammann G, Riemenschneider A, Walter M, et al: The impact of interpersonal problems in borderline personality disorder patients on treatment outcome and psychotherapy. Psychopathology 49(3):172–180, 2016

Dulz B, Lohmer M, Kernberg OF, et al: Borderline-Persönlichkeitsstörung: Übertragungs-Fokussierte Psychotherpie. Göttingen, Germany, Hogrefe, 2021

Ezriel H: A psychoanalytic approach to the treatment of patients in groups. J Ment Sci 96:774–779, 1950

Fairbairn WD: An Object-Relations Theory of the Personality. New York, Basic Books, 1952

Foulkes SH, Anthony EJ: Group Psychotherapy: The Psychoanalytic Approach. Baltimore, MD, Penguin, 1957

Häfner S, Lieberz K, Hölzer M, Wöller W: Wann kommt ihr patient in die klinik? Indikationen für die stationäre psychotherapie. MMW-Fortschritt der Medizin 43:28–31, 2001

Jones M: The Therapeutic Community: A New Treatment Method in Psychiatry. New York, Basic Books, 1953

Kernberg OF: Ideology, Conflict and Leadership in Groups and Organizations. New Haven, CT, Yale University Press, 1998

Kernberg OF: Psychoanalytic individual and group psychotherapy: the transference-focused psychotherapy (TFP) model, in The Inseparable Nature of Love and Aggression: Clinical and Theoretical Perspectives. Edited by Kernberg OF. Washington, DC, American Psychiatric Publishing, 2012, pp 31–55

Klein M: Notes on some schizoid mechanisms, in Developments in Psychoanalysis. Edited by Klein M, Heiman P, Isaacs S, Riviere J. London, Hogarth, 1946, pp 202–320

Linehan MM: Cognitive Behavioral Treatment of Borderline Personality Disorder. New York, Guilford, 1993

Main TF: The hospital as a therapeutic institution. Bull Menninger Clin 10:66–70, 1946

Main TF: The ailment. Br J Med Psychol 30:129–145, 1957

Plakun EM: Treatment Resistance and Patient Authority: The Austen Riggs Reader. New York, Norton, 2011

Rice AK: The Enterprise and Its Environment. London, Tavistock, 1963

Rice AK: Learning for Leadership. London, Tavistock, 1965

Rice AK: Individual group and intergroup processes. Human Relations 22:565–584, 1969

Rioch MJ: Group relations: rationale and technique. Int J Group Psychother 10:340–355, 1970a

Rioch MJ: The work of Wilfred Bion on groups. Psychiatry 33:56–66, 1970b

Rosenfeld H: Notes on the psychoanalysis of the super-ego conflict in an acute schizophrenia patient, in Psychotherapy of Schizophrenia and Manic-Depressive States. Edited by Azima H, Glueck BC. Washington, DC, American Psychiatric Association, 1955

Sollberger D, Gremaud-Heitz D, Riemenschneider A, et al: Change in self functioning and psychopathology in patients with borderline personality disorder during TFP-based disorder-specific inpatient treatment: a prospective, controlled study over 12 weeks. Clin Psychol Psychother 22(6):559–569, 2014

Stanton AM, Schwartz M: The Mental Hospital. New York, Basic Books, 1954

Sullivan HS: Conceptions of Modern Psychiatry. New York, 1953a

Sullivan HS: The Interpersonal Theory of Psychiatry. New York, Norton, 1953b

Sutherland JD: Notes on psychoanalytic group therapy, I: therapy and training. Psychiatry 15:111–117, 1952

Yeomans FE, Clarkin JF, Kernberg OF: Transference-Focused Psychotherapy for Borderline Personality Disorder: A Clinical Guide. Washington, DC, American Psychiatric Publishing, 2015

CHAPTER 11

Malignant Narcissism and Large Group Regression

From a psychoanalytic perspective, we have to recognize that a psychoanalytic understanding only covers a limited area of the complex social forces triggered by the interaction of regressed large groups and the corresponding pathological leadership: the nature of historical determinants of the formation of social subgroups; the origin of cultural, social, political, religious, and social bias; the cause of present traumatic circumstances; and the political system within which regressed large groups consolidate are important determinants that influence the development of such leadership–followers' constellations. Does psychoanalytic understanding have anything to say about whether and how we can use our present-day understanding to help prevent such calamitous situations in the future?

The purpose of this paper is to analyze the mutual relationships between large group regression and the emergence of a particular kind of leadership related to that regressive process, namely, leaders with characteristics of the syndrome of malignant narcissism. The main hypothesis to be explored is that the nature of large group regression translates into the search for that particular personality type—and that personalities with the syndrome of malignant narcissism are prone to aspire to leadership and are very effective in achieving leadership of the regressed large group under these conditions. The mutual influence of the culture of the regressed large group and its corresponding ideological development and the characteristic behaviors of a leader evincing malignant narcissism stimulates typical behaviors in the leader. In turn, the corresponding leadership reinforces some basic characteristics of regressed large groups. To explore that linkage, we shall review briefly the concept of regression in group processes, studying group psychology both in large groups and "mass" psychology, and in small groups, reviewing the relevant contributions by Freud, Bion, Turquet, Volkan, and others. This review will be followed by the exploration of the preferred personality structures of leadership fostered by these different group structures, and the relationship between functional leadership and pathological leadership related to the requirements expressed in group regression. I then shall summarize briefly the syndrome of malignant narcissism and its derivative leadership characteristics in social institutions and the political process at large.

Psychoanalytic Group Psychology

Freud, in his 1921 text on "Group Psychology and the Analysis of the Ego" outlined what became one of the most original and tragically relevant contributions to the study of the dynamic unconscious, namely, the behavior of what in German is called "masse" (Freud 1921/1949). It refers to mass movements, or large conglomerates of people united by a common ideal, a common sense of identity related to race, religion, nationality, or a particular ideology that unifies this enormous conglomerate of individuals in an active direction or cohesive move under the direction of a particular leader. This mass psychology has to be differentiated from the situation of crowds, that is, the accidental getting together of an enormous number of people as part of usual social interactions, without any common direction or sense of a specific mutual relationship. Freud described political mass movements, particularly of fascism and communism, years before the common characteristics of mass movements and their consequences had been experienced dramatically, as it evolved in the 20th and now in the 21st century.

Freud pointed out that the individual who senses himself as part of such a mass movement acquires a reduced capacity for independent judgment and rational decision-making. To the contrary, what dominates the individuals within the mass movement is a sense of power by mutual identification, a sense of belonging and power derived from being part of such a large movement. It is their mutual identification that coincides with their identification with the leader of the mass movement, which provides them with a sense of shared identity, an identification with the leader who is not only powerful and idealized but also feared. At the same time, he assumes consciously and in the mind of his followers the responsibility for the direction of the movement and frees all the individuals from themselves having to make decisions about that movement. More generally, mass psychology induces the projection onto the leader of the individuals' ego ideal, so that moral consciousness is projected onto the leader and the individuals in the mass feel free from moral constraints. They acquire a degree of freedom that goes together with a characteristic activation of intense affective dispositions shared by the entire mass and is particularly of an aggressive, destructive type, the target of which is directed outside the mass movement. As part of mass psychology, the participants feel powerful and secure and united in the free, unconstrained, and personally irresponsible participation in aggression against outside, feared, hated, and depreciated groups who are perceived as threatening the mass movement. The shared sense of equality, power, and freedom from moral constraints is the counterpart to a heightened suggestibility to the commands from the leader, a suggestibility enhanced by the decrease of rational, independent judgment induced by the psychology of the mass movement.

Wilfred Bion's (1961) analysis of the relation between groups and their leadership introduced a new method of psychoanalytic exploration of group psychology. As a courageous and effective tank commander in the First World War, and in his later work as a psychiatrist in military psychiatric hospitals and War Office Selection Boards during the Second World War, he developed professional experiences with both effective task groups and regressed, demoralized ones, and their leadership. He combined his psychoanalytic training and Tavistock Clinic experience, the application of Kleinian concepts of splitting and projective identification in individual treatments with his group studies and experiences in what became a new field of psychoanalytic inquiry.

Bion's (1961) studies of small group psychology provided a complementary analysis of the intimate processes affecting the regression of individuals when they are part of a group process. He described the behavior evolving in small groups of 10–15 members that were exclusively engaged in observing their own experiences and behavior in limited time sessions from 1–2 hours. He observed typical developments that he described as the "basic assumptions groups" of "dependency," "fight-flight," and "pairing." These "basic assumptions" groups emerged typically and consistently when such a small group had no specific task that would justify its existence and link it with an environment by a concrete objective that has to be accomplished. A group that gets together with a task of learning a determined subject, developing a particular project, or constructing particular objects represents "work groups" that operate rationally and with a realistic organization of the development of the particular group task. When such a task does not exist and the only group task is the observation of the group itself and the emotional consequences of such a lack of a specific task, then the basic assumptions emerge.

The basic assumption of "dependency" is characterized by a general sense of insecurity, uncertainty, and immaturity on the part of members of the group, who look for a leader who will help them understand their situation, direct the group, provide their needs, feed them with knowledge, meaning, or security, a leader who presents self-assurance and an attitude of potency and knowledge that is supportive and reassuring, provokes his idealization by the group, and the wish to depend on him. Competition for becoming the preferred "child" of that leader, mutual jealousy for the amount of attention each member of the group gets from their idealized leader, illustrates the fact that this self-assured, knowledgeable, giving leader provides a sense of safety and security in being part of the group. In contrast, fear and insecurity develop if one falls outside the assured membership of such a group. If the leader does not provide the assurance of the gratification of the group's dependency needs, the members of the group experience strong disappointment or disillusionment, search for an alternative leader in the group who may replace him, idealize the new leader while attributing to him the attributes they had seen in the previous leader, and expect him to carry out the needed function of leadership of the dependent group.

The situation in the basic assumption group of "fight-flight" is completely different. Here there is a sense of tension and conflict, a preparedness to fight against out-groups, and a sense of group unity as part of this fighting disposition against out-groups. Sometimes, when there is no such evident adversary out-group, a division of the very group evolves into an "in-group" who stands with the leader and an "out-group" that fights the leader and the in-group. The search here is for a strong, self-righteous, distrustful, and controlling leader who provides leadership in the struggle with the enemy out-group or the rebellious subgroup. In contrast to the predominance, in the dependent group, of mechanisms of primitive idealization, regressive dependency, and denial of all conflicts around authority issues, here, in the fight-flight group, there is a remarkable development of splitting operations between "us" and "them," the in-group and the out-group, a sharp differentiation between idealization of the in-group and projection of aggression and attacks on the out-group, and a tendency to submit to the leader as part of the psychology of a shared sense of discipline required by the fight against assumed enemies. Splitting, projective identification, and denial of aggression within the internal subgroup go hand in hand with the search for a leader who will gratify the need for this organization, usually a powerful individual with paranoid features who fits the group's demand for a sharp division between the ideal inner world of the group and a dangerous threatening external world that needs to be fought off.

In the "pairing" group, finally, a still different atmosphere prevails. Here the group selects a couple, heterosexual or homosexual, that the group perceives as united, bound together by mutual identification, love, and commitment. The group admires the couple because it corresponds to the wish for establishing such an ideal couple love relationship, an ideal shared by all the members and expressed in this idealization but also in the related need to fight off envious feelings about this selected ideal couple. There is a sexual quality in the air, an erotized quality of relations that differs from both the regressed dependent relations of the dependent group and from the tense, aggressive challenging and distrustful atmosphere of the fight-flight group. While the dependent group preferably selects a leader with strong narcissistic features, the fight-flight group selects a leader with paranoid features, and the pairing group a leader who tolerates the development of such a pair, helps to protect it, and conveys the assurance to the group that the erotic quality of the development of intimate relations is tolerated and welcome. The "pairing" group represents a less regressive, "oedipal" group experience.

Within the growing interest in developing Bion's approach to groups at the Tavistock Clinic, Pierre Turquet's (1975) work stands out. With a related background in military medical services to Bion's, Turquet expanded the study of regressed group behavior to larger family groups and social institutions, and, in following Bion's approach, he carried out empirical work with larger groups. He studied the behavior of large groups. These were experimental groups of 100–300 members, also gathered only to study the nature of their experiences and behavior over a period of a 1.5–2 hours, with the provision of a group leader. This leader, similarly to the leader provided to small groups, limits himself or herself to comment on dominant emotional experiences shared by the group without assuming the particular leadership functions demanded by the group. The small groups establish by themselves particular expectations from the leader, once they are clearly in the dependent, fight-flight, or pairing position; the "professional" group leader will not gratify but analyze their emotional needs. Thus, the leaders that have been described for the small groups are selected and seduced into their respective leadership function in terms of the corresponding psychology of the respective small group. A similar phenomenon happens in the large group. The large group, usually, as I mentioned, composed of a membership between 100 and a maximum of 300 persons, gets together in concentric circles that permit the members of still seeing each other and responding to each other—similarly as in the small group, but evidently this situation reduces enormously the possibility of the constitution of cohesive, small subgroups. All the individuals of the large group are much more isolated from each other than is the case of small group psychology.

The large group meets without any particular task except to experience and discuss its own developments. Every member has the right to speak up at any moment, and the professional group leader limits himself/herself to observing, from time to time, the dominant emotional issues affecting the group. The leader does not organize the development of any subject of the group discussions at any point. Here, again, if the large group were "structured," organized to carry out a certain task, for example, to discuss or decide about a particular subject around which it would establish an order or procedure of order and time limitations within which individuals can speak up, this would transform the group into a "work group" and become realistically focused on and occupied with such a task. The unstructured large group, to the contrary, is totally open to whatever anybody in the group may feel like saying or doing.

The typical development in such large group situations is an enormous sense of loss of personal identity, as the individual in it cannot reliably find a commonality with anybody else. In the large group situation, efforts emerge to establish subgroups on the basis of whatever members may try to find as commonalities: needs, language, religion, profession, political views, race, or appearance of any kind; but these efforts usually fail, and the group develops rapidly a collective sense of intense anxiety. While people speak freely, there is a tendency not to listen to what other people are saying. Individuals who speak up obtain no feedback. Clear efforts at projective identification fail because of the difficulty to focus on and control the reactions of others to oneself. There is a general sense of impotence and fearfulness that develops in the members, and a fear of aggression to explode in the group. At times the group is able to identify a small subgroup within the large group or outside it and gather around a joined, intense hate reaction against such a subgroup. This, temporarily transforms the large group into a small mass that fights an external enemy, but even such efforts usually fail.

A tendency develops in the group for individuals to emerge that are trying to analyze rationally what is happening. It is characteristic for the large group that particularly intelligent, self-reflective, rational people are shut down immediately. To the contrary, naïve, cliché formulating individuals who have a simplistic statement to make tend to be supported, with a slightly derogatory, amused attitude, by the group at large but, at the same time, with a shared sense of relief, and such cliché spreading mediocrities are preferentially selected as leader of the large group. The group conveys the impression that there is a shared envy of individuals who maintain their individuality, security, rationality, and, with such a capacity, attempt to provide group leadership, while there is support of a mediocre leadership that reassures everybody and provides a calming sense of security, while at the same time there is a shared subtle devaluation of that selected leader.

As an alternative development, if the intensity of anxiety and aggressive feelings is excessive, the group may veer into a paranoid direction. It selects a paranoid individual who finds a cause to fight against, a group or an intolerable social condition, something in the external world which everybody agrees needs to be fought against and potentially destroyed. Thus, the large group, at the bottom, oscillates between the search for a narcissistic leader with a nonthreatening, simplistic quality that can be depreciated and promises a tranquilizing passivity, or else, under activation of an excessive degree of aggression, a powerful paranoid leader who unifies the group into a fighting attitude that transforms the large group into a small "mass psychology" group as described by Freud.

Vamik Volkan (2004) has expanded greatly our understanding of group psychology with what he refers to as large group regression but what has to be differentiated from the large group as originally described by Turquet (1975) and others. Both Bion and Turquet studied artificial groups, brought together for the purpose of observing group behavior. Volkan's work focuses on the study of naturally occurring groups, especially in times of crisis. Volkan, in fact, refers to mass psychology in the sense of Freud's analysis of the psychology of large conglomerates united by a sense of mutual cohesiveness, equality, and fraternity and a common set of ideas—a common ideology—that expresses their unifying disposition, including the potential relationship to an idealized, feared, and/or direction signaling leader. Volkan studied group psychological behavior in international conflicts and conflicts between nationalistic or religious opposite political groups, and, particularly, the psychological developments related to the traumatic effects of the terrorist attack in New York on September 11, 2001.

In summary, Volkan proposes that, under conditions of traumatic situations, social revolutions, nature caused disasters, economic crisis, and, generally speaking, the collapse of traditional cultural structures that regulate the daily life of the individual, the strong possibility of a large group regression develops, within which the normal social structure that assures the individual of his status—role relationships—disappears. Under such conditions, there evolves a threat to normal identity that ordinarily is reinforced by the status and role conditions of every individual within this social and cultural environment. There now evolves a search for a "second skin," a new external social structure that returns the security that had protected individual identity and sense of security. Here the emergence of a large group leader becomes important in providing to the social group in crisis a voice that reconfirms their commonality, the sense of a common ideology that assures the large group of its basic existential security, historical mission, and goodness and differentiates it from external enemies or enemy situations that had been threatening it. The leader calls for joint action to stand up and, in short, provides the large group with a new sense of identity in terms of all the individuals belonging to that mass movement.

There is a tendency of a large group in an existential social crisis to rally blindly around such a leader, who eliminates the traditional status and role relations of individuals derived mostly from their belonging to a family, to specific relations to family members, and to the social group related to it. The leader creates a new collective "family" structure in terms of the historical importance and mission of the group. The community becomes divided into a "good" segment (the large group) that obediently follows the leader and a "bad" segment of those perceived as opposing the leader. A sharp division between "us" and "them" is established, and "them" become enemies that need to be fought off, defended against, and attacked. The large group develops a sense of shared morality of the "good" system that becomes increasingly absolutist and punitive toward those who are in conflict with it, and the group may experience periods of massive mood swings from shared depressed feelings over the nature of the critical or dramatic situation that originated the present situation to collective paranoid projection of aggression towards outsiders. The sense of internal goodness becomes a sense of entitlement and a gradual distortion of reality in which unpleasant and threatening aspects of reality are denied. There evolve new cultural phenomena or modified versions of traditional social customs with particular focus on joint traumas and past triumphs of the group residing in a time collapse in which past and present is confused. The leadership feeds into this collapse of the time perspective by creating a break in the actual historical continuity of the group and filling the gap with a "new" nationalism, a new shared sentience or a "new" morality, and a transformation of the actual history of the group.

The large group members begin to experience shared symbols as "protosymbols," including shared images that depict enemy groups with symbols or protosymbols associated with bodily waste, vermin, dangerous or toxic animal traits. The large group consolidates its unity by erecting sharp boundaries with the outside world, focusing on minor differences between itself and enemy groups, and searches powerfully for commonalities in its natural condition, origin, and convictions as part of their new "second skin" that protects its identity. The large group may initiate behaviors that symbolize its purification. It may change its attitude towards aesthetics, to what is considered beautiful and ugly, and there is a tendency for the large group to turn the physical environment into an amorphous gray-brown (fecal or decomposing) structure. All these characteristics constitute an ideologically fundamented, consolidated, and expressively lived activation of the clear, separate "second skin" identity that provides the combination of security, power, freedom, moral superiority, and irresponsibility described by Freud for mass psychology. Volkan's analysis enriches and bridges the analysis of large group psychology by Turquet with Freud's analysis of mass psychology.

The combined analysis of group regression, from small group regression to large group regression and to mass psychology, illustrates some basic commonalities of these various processes. The motive for group regression, in all cases, is a loss of the functional relationship of individuals within a stable, small or large social and cultural structure. This social and cultural structure is given by an ordinary living situation within a stable social environment not threatened by major political, international, or economic catastrophes or nature determined calamities. And, in the case of small groups, the loss of the functional tasks of the group by design or other circumstances replicates temporarily that loss of functional stability of the individual. This loss of the traditional social structure signifies a threat to individual identity, and it signals the extent to which normal identity function is supported and assured by the individual's psychosocial environment. Massive loss of such a protective environment that simultaneously affects a selected group or an entire community leads to powerful anxiety and initiates regressive functions.

It is significant that the anxiety, in all cases, has to do with a threat of a definite experience of danger, the activation of negative, aggressive affect states and correspondent defensive operations that we know from the study of severe psychopathology of individuals with primitive aggressive aggression dominated conflicts. These defensive operations, particularly splitting mechanisms, projective identification, denial, primitive idealization and devaluation, omnipotent control—all of them described by Melanie Klein (1946) as characteristic of the paranoid-schizoid position—emerge in the dependent and fight-flight group, where they structure the group within the given basic assumptions orientation, but they are ineffective for the individual in the large group situation. Here the only effective protection is an individual's isolating himself from the large group situation into the position of a "singleton" (Turquet 1975), which will coincide with a sense of impotence and alienation and the loss of participation in the social process. The large majority caught up in the activation of massive paranoid-schizoid defenses of the large group will participate in a joint effort to compensate for the loss of individual identity by the collective search for leadership to replace individual identity by the "second skin" described by Volkan. In other words, it is a search for a new, shared identity linked to the dependency of a particular type of leadership. The type of leadership selected will oscillate between the narcissistic type of leader, as in the dependent group and the large narcissistic group described by Turquet, or a paranoid leader, as in the fight-flight group, in the mass movement or in the large group described by Turquet when intense aggression overrides the reassuring search for a narcissistic, calming leader. I have described in earlier work (Kernberg 1998) how the nature of the ideology selected by the large group, particularly in mass movements, also oscillates between a narcissistic and a paranoid type. Many political and religious ideologies contain a central, humanistic core that, under different conditions of group regression, may shift into a paranoid or a narcissistic distortion of the ideology. Moscovici (1981), in his sociological analysis of the effects of media and mass communication, has suggested that, while Marx described religion as the "opium of the people," the media and mass communication are the "Valium" of the people.

Leadership and Malignant Narcissism

In earlier analyses of the characteristics of functional leadership of social organizations, I pointed out that essential qualities of functional leadership include the following: 1) high intelligence, possibly best defined by the time span of decision making (Jacques 1976), that is, the capacity of leadership to foresee long-time developments and orient the organization he or she leads in the light of this analysis; 2) an integrated personality structure that includes the capacity for significant self-reflection and assessment in depth of other people, essential to selecting delegate leadership and deciding about conflicts that involve technical knowledge as well as personality features; 3) a solid, autonomous moral capacity and commitment, given the unavoidable corruptive temptations of leadership functions; 4) significant narcissistic features—in the sense of solid security and self-regard that permit leadership to tolerate the unavoidable ambivalences and aggression stemming from the internal functioning of the organization as well as from external sources of challenges to it; 5) a sufficient availability of paranoid traits—in the sense of a mature distrust in contrast to naiveté that would ignore aggressive and potentially threatening developments in the work relationships of the organization.

A discrete, reasonable and controlled amount of narcissistic and paranoid features are an important aspect of leadership, in contrast to excessive dependence needs that cannot be gratified outside the leadership function and a dangerous naiveté regarding the complexity of human relations in social organizations. Precisely these two personality features, in an exaggerated and pathological way, typically characterize the leaders selected in regressive group situations, problematic organizational functioning, and mass movements. From a different perspective, Canetti (1960) described the psychological characteristics of the "feasting mass," (*festmasse*), and the "hounding mass" (*hetzmasse*). These refer to the predominant behavior of respectively celebrating narcissistically or aggressively persecuting large groups under the corresponding leadership of a narcissistic and potentially hypomanic leader organizing collective feasts and orgies, in contrast to the paranoid leader of an aggressive, persecutory mob. In short, an extraordinary potential for narcissistic or paranoid leadership emerges under conditions of large group regression.

At this point, we have to explore the nature of narcissistic and paranoid character traits that are characteristic, respectively, of narcissistic and paranoid personality disorders. In fact, under conditions of social disorganization, the weakening of traditional social structures, the emergence of extremist political groups and parties, individuals with these characteristics tend to become important in providing a "second skin" to the respective groups. But there is one type of particularly relevant psychopathology that combines narcissistic and paranoid traits as part of a severe type of narcissistic personality disorder, namely, the syndrome of malignant narcissism.

I have defined the syndrome of malignant narcissism in earlier studies of severe forms of pathological narcissism (Kernberg 1984, 2018) as characterized by the presence of 1) a narcissistic personality disorder with all its characteristic features: a pathological grandiose self, inordinate self-centeredness and a sense of superiority, strong manifestations of envy, devaluation of others, severe limitations of the capacity of emotional investment in others, and a chronic sense of emptiness that requires an ongoing search for external stimulation or the excitement derived from drugs or sexual behavior; 2) significant paranoid personality features; 3) strong ego-syntonic aggression directed against others or self, and 4) significant antisocial behavior. The basic psychopathological features of the syndrome of malignant narcissism are a dominance of unconscious conflicts around intense aggressive affect—from whatever origin, together with the development of the compensating pathology of a grandiose self. Aggressive motivation infiltrates the grandiose sense of self, leading to ego-syntonic aggressivity on the one hand and to the projection of aggression in the form of paranoid tendencies on the other. The severe deficit in the development of an internalized system of ethical values derived from the underlying basic failure in normal identity formation that affects the buildup of such an ethical structure (superego development) determines the development of antisocial behaviors.

Patients with the syndrome of malignant narcissism function along a wide spectrum of social dysfunction. The most ill patients with these characteristics suffer from a total breakdown of their capacity for social interactions, incapacity to function in work and profession, and breakdown in intimate relations, together with the development of severe affective dysregulation, and such a degree of disturbed interpersonal behavior that makes for initial confusion with borderline personality disorder. At the other extreme are patients who are able to maintain their social functions and work conditions and only show breakdown in their personal, intimate relationships, an incapacity to significantly invest in nonexploitive behavior with others, and an extremely exaggerated concept of self and commitment to self-interests that are pursued in an aggressive way without moral restrictions. It so happens that such individuals may be perfectly adaptable to a social situation of massive group regression, in which these aspects of their personality function effectively to gratify basic needs of the regressed large group.

Under ordinary circumstances, such relatively well functioning individuals presenting malignant narcissism, possessing high intelligence, unusual technical capabilities, and knowledge in some specialized area and the capability to fulfill their ambitions to promotion within social organizations, may assume leadership of social organizations in education, health, military, and religious institutions or industry. They usually promote the institution by identifying their personal interests with that of the institution, but, over a period of time, because of their severe incapacity to assess others, their tendency to surround themselves with adulating subordinates, and their incapacity to tolerate criticism and therefore use realistic, essential feedback for institutional operations, such institutions show a typical regression. The organization evolves a sharp differentiation of levels of emotional climates. At the top of the organization, surrounding the leadership with malignant narcissism, are individuals who also present narcissistic and antisocial features. They have learned to adjust themselves to the needs of the leader to be both loved and feared while being unaffected by his interpersonal demandingness and, at times, antisocial maneuvers, so leadership with antisocial features expands corruption at the top. At a second level of organizational functioning, including the large majority of professional and institutional staff, there develops an intensely paranoid atmosphere because of the fear of a leader who is hypersensitive to criticism, who needs to be shown love and admiration, and who cannot listen to anything running against his or her will. There is a high level of institutional "paranoiagenesis" (Jacques 1976), with frequent turnover and breakdown of staff. At the bottom level of the institution, at the periphery of its internal emotional milieu, one finds the most capable staff members, depressed and alienated, prone to be the first ones to leave the organization, sometimes depriving an organization of the most productive and creative members of its staff. So far, I summarized what happens in organized social institutions.

Large Group Regression and Malignant Narcissistic Leadership

In contrast to the developments in well-structured social organizations, under conditions of social disorganization and large group regression, the emergence of leaders with the syndrome of malignant narcissism takes further, socially dysfunctional and threatening characteristics. The leader's narcissistic self-centeredness and grandiosity, his self-assured signaling what he believes the large group should think and do, and his promise for a brilliant future if he is followed powerfully reassures the members of a regressed large group against the threat of the loss of individual identity and provides them with the second skin of an idealizing mutual identity of all in identification with the leader. The reduced cognitive level of functioning characteristic of large groups (Kernberg 1998; Turquet 1975) responds positively to simple slogans and clichés that the leader provides them with to confirm their value, uniqueness, importance, and power. Simple slogans replace complex thinking and correspond to the large group's need to feel that they are intimately involved with the thinking of the great leader and understand him completely, and, at a deeper, unconscious level, don't need to envy him. Everybody is equal in the pursuit of simple ideals and in the proper symbolic expression of such ideas. The well rationalized aggression against out-groups is fostered by the leader's direct, crude, and sadistic expression of animosity against such out-groups, devaluing and dehumanizing them while declaring the large group he directs to be the selected, ideal, morally justified, superior social group. Aggressive outbursts against minorities is fostered, welcome, considered heroic and morally admirable, so that freedom to express destructive behavior excites the group and creates a contaminating festive atmosphere. Bao-Lord (1990) describes how, during the Chinese Cultural Revolution, the beating up of professors by revolutionary groups in the middle of huge public gatherings contaminated the bystanders so that massive engagement in physical attack and murder became a welcome public spectacle.

The characteristic antisocial features of the leader with malignant narcissism are reflected in practically public dishonest behavior, matched with shameless denial of that behavior. Hitler never acknowledged his clear, indirect instructions to eliminate potentially rivalrous leaders of his S.A. troops; he never acknowledged publicly, nor in writing, his instructions for mass murder of the Jewish population under his control, in spite of being the obvious ultimate source of these orders. Stalin would invite both privileged followers whom he wished to honor for tea at his place and also those who already had been secretly condemned to be eliminated. This was sufficiently well known in his intimate circle to cause extreme anxiety in the invitees, which, apparently, greatly pleased Stalin.

The leader's evident dishonesty, the self-assured expression of lies that may be easily recognized as such by an outside observer and a broader social environment or general community, is perceived by the regressed large group as a courageous standing up to conventional truth, daring to say the impossible, the leader showing courage in changing his mind at any point and shifting over, if necessary, to declaring alternative choices of who is the selected enemy at the moment. The leader's decidedly assuming moral responsibility promotes a sense of freedom from moral constraints, excitement of moving with a powerful wave of political discontent and strife as it is manipulated from the top and cemented by the suggestibility of the large group. Repeated attacks, ridiculing, and demeaning humiliation of selected "enemies" reinforce the group's enjoyment of sadistic behavior. It was the inhumane cruelty of ISIS that exerted an exciting attractiveness to many early international followers.

Leadership by a leader with malignant narcissism within an institutional, task oriented organization is circumscribed by the very structure of the organization; the need to carry out its technical or professional functions, the outside world that confronts the organization with consequences of failure of leadership in carrying out ordinary boundary functions, in addition to the negative effects of decreased productivity and deterioration of human relations in the inside of such an organization. External authorities, Board of Governors, or community oversight tends to limit, in the long run, the negative effects of deficient leadership. In an open, political field, in contrast, the negative consequences of the mutual stimulation between large group regression and the emergence of leadership with malignant narcissistic personality characteristics is much more effective in its destructive consequences.

To begin with, the crystallization of a regressed social subgroup, that is, the constitution of a large group with shared feelings of threatening insecurity related to economic, cultural, or political issues, with threats to the identity or survival of that group, is experienced and shared informally by the group. A general feeling of growing tension, anxiety, and irritability initiates the search for a "second skin," that is, a longed for, decisive intervention by leadership to protect the well-being, security, and stability of the group's existence. The situation is open now to a self-assured, aggressive, powerful combative politician who spells out the generally shared feelings of dissatisfaction and resentment and orients the group toward an external source of its troubles in the form of an external enemy power that needs to be fought off. A general paranoid orientation evolves and consolidates the large group in the active search, identification, and separation from the designated enemy group. The cultural availability of a preexisting ideology with strongly paranoid features, or one that can be shifted easily into a paranoid direction, may be used by a leader to establish a sense of historical continuity of this struggle with adversary forces and include historical trauma and triumphs to provide a sense of mission in the direction of restoring such past glory or undoing historical trauma, creating a dynamic force in the pursuit of justice and right (Volkan 2004).

The antisocial potential of the leader with malignant narcissism may manifest itself at first only in relatively discrete dishonest behaviors, such as evident lies, false accusations, and circumscribed distortions of reality, all of which is expressed, however, in a courageous way that implicitly tests the extent to which the community at large may threaten the specific regressed large group with creating limits to this dishonesty or accept it. As Turquet (1975) had originally pointed out, and is also stressed by Albright (2018) and Snyder (2017), there is a "third group" constituted by the original total population that watches a combative minority—the large regressed group—enter into warfare with another social subgroup, the selected victims of the attacks by the dynamic, regressed large group possessed by an extreme, paranoid ideology. If the traditional structure of society is weakened by a present traumatic situation, an economic crisis, a lost war, a natural disaster, the initial response to the provocative dishonesty that the leadership of the regressed large group propagates may be sufficiently weak, and ordinary social reactions not sufficiently alarmed to stand up against such a distortion in social communication. Now more destructive aggressive acts, distortion of reality, open encouragement of violence may develop, with an expanding affirmation and dissemination of the certainty, self-righteousness, the sense of moral justification and superiority emanating from the revolutionary large group under the stimulation by the leader. The aggressive, paranoid, and dishonest behavior socially fostered by malignant narcissistic leadership thus evolves into an ever-growing sense of self-confirmation and power by the group. The self-assuredness of the leader and the expansion of his paranoid, grandiose, and aggressive behavior go hand in hand with the increase of a sense of power, freedom, violent behavior, and triumphant excitement of the regressed large group.

The Dangers to Society

Jacques Semelin (2007) illustrates all these processes with the initial anti-Semitic ideology, work restrictions, and media attacks on Jews in Nazi Germany during the early stages of the Hitler regime, and their gradual escalation as initial resistance against social acts of violence was muted, and a gradual increase in physical violence, socially destructive behavior, and arbitrary legislation restricting Jewish life and robbing Jewish property was calmly accepted by the German population at large. In general, at this stage, relatively independent social structures, particularly, religious organizations, the armed forces, the financial elite, the judicial power, the media, the strength of bureaucratic organization, and tradition become important elements that may control this regressive process or reinforce it. The combined influence of these relatively stable social structures and powers may then determine the extent to which a regressive process evolves further into the potential extreme of the development of genocidal regimes, or is controlled in the form of an ordinary dictatorship, or ends with the eventual recovery of the civilized reaction to this social regression. An independent military that traditionally rejects its identification with a particular political orientation may counteract the establishment of a totalitarian regime, that is, an effort by the malignant narcissistic leadership to establish an obligatory indoctrination of the entire population by a determined ideological doctrine.

It needs to be stressed that totalitarian systems differ from ordinary dictatorships in their imposition of an obligatory ideological system. You don't only have to fear the leader but also must love him. The totalitarian regime established by personalities with malignant narcissism will be reinforced by such an ideology centered on the idealization and fearful submission to the leader, but an ordinary dictatorship, while less effective, also tends to achieve the same submission and destructive effects on the population. The surprising reaction of the military establishment of the Soviet Union in dropping its allegiance to the communist party happened at a point when the economic failure of the communist system interfered with the effective military competition with the United States. This development contributed fundamentally to the downfall of the communist regime. To the contrary, the German military fell rapidly into place with Nazi ideology, given its crucial role in the expansionist doctrine of national-socialist ideology geared to establish the dominance of Germany over Europe.

Social media may express an identification with a dominant traditional culture that rejects the extremes that threaten a peaceful coexistence of different ideological orientations and break the expansionist power of a revolutionary extreme group. The very fact that the Internet permits the parallel diffusion, circulation, and expansion of completely contradictory ideological investments may protect a democratic political system, but it may also be used by extremist social subgroups to organize a hidden rebellion against the status quo and facilitate communication of regressed large groups, as has been illustrated by the effective recruitment tool that the Internet has signified for terrorist Islamic groups in recent times.

In general, once a totalitarian power achieves control of the media, they become an important instrument of social indoctrination. An independent judicial system may be a significant counterweight to the aggressive assault on individual's rights and invasion of individual privacy by revolutionary groups with totalitarian ideology. But when a revolutionary government is able to control ordinary judiciary power, laws and judges may easily become corrupt. An effective bureaucracy may prevent, to some extent, social disorganization and the disruption of ordinary interactions of individuals and institutions, but a highly organized bureaucracy under state control may powerfully reinforce a totalitarian system.

A dramatic overall comparative study of genocide in three very different societies carried out by Jacques Semelin (2007) illustrates the worst-case scenarios of progression of social regression of large groups with corresponding malignant narcissistic leadership into mass murder and genocide. He compares the historical developments of Rwanda, Bosnia, and Nazi Germany leading to genocidal explosion and reaches the conclusion that similar processes occurred in all three so very different societies in terms of the historical background, culture, and sociopolitical situation. In all three cases a latent animosity existed between social subgroups, Tutsi and Hutu in Rwanda, Muslims and Christians in Bosnia, the historical anti-Semitism of German culture and its rejection of the Jews. Such latent potential social splits became expressed first in all three cases in a general ideological disposition, an extreme ideology turning one group against the other. That divisive ideology became acute at the time of social crisis derived from the complexities of decolonization in the case of Rwanda, the aftermath of the decomposition of the communist system in Yugoslavia, the consequence of the defeat of the First World War and the later economic crisis in Germany. This led to the ascent of leadership by personalities with powerful aggressive, paranoid, and antisocial features, who started out with grandiose leadership aspirations in all three cases. The end result of this process was a totalitarian situation with a socially imposed, ideologically rationalized, leadership supported political program called to exterminate the enemy group. We have more detailed information, at this point, of both Hitler's and Stalin's personalities that documents the pathology of malignant narcissism in both of them. It refers to their extraordinary grandiosity, the savage aggression and personal sadistic pleasure in torturing their enemies, their dishonesty and paranoia, and the strange incapacity to evaluate the personality features of their immediate secondary leadership. It is no coincidence that Hitler felt closest to the two most similar personalities to himself in terms of grandiosity and dishonesty, Goebbels and Goering, and Stalin ended up trusting the psychopathic Beria more than any other member of his leadership group.

When the ascent of groups with the characteristics of regressed large group psychology, and of corresponding leadership with features of malignant narcissism is socially limited in its size, effectiveness, durability, and dramatic impact on the corresponding surrounding society, such a group may emerge as a religious or political cult that ends up in self-destruction or control by the wider social community and state. Obviously, those cults leading to murder or collective suicide represent extremes of this pathology.

In earlier work (Kernberg 2003) discussing the prevention of socially sanctioned violence, I focused on the limited tools available from a psychoanalytic viewpoint and expertise, including a focused attention on childhood neglect and violence and the corresponding interventions at the home, in early infant and child care, in the school, and the conscious effort to combat and prevent cultural bias with active, socially fostered measures against racial, political, sexual, religious, and other ideologically tinged prejudices against social subgroups. I also questioned the concept of multi-culturalism in terms of its fostering the coexistence of sharply different subcultures within the same social environment. I stressed the need that particularly immigrants from a different culture be helped to integrate into the culture of a country in which they are making their new home. So far, we have studied how we can contribute to reduce the burden of social prejudice against subgroups: concerted efforts of the educational approach in elementary and high school may be an important corrective. Regarding the selection of leadership, in social organizations as well as in political systems, I believe that we are progressing somewhat in the awareness of the psychological requirements of good leadership that may be considered in the selection not only of institutional leadership but, perhaps even more importantly, in the evaluation of potential political leadership. But this awareness does not assure the utilization and effectiveness of this knowledge.

The selection of good leadership in social organizations with clear boundaries, defined tasks, and correspondent administrative structures is realistically feasible. Usually leaders are selected who evince appropriate technical knowledge and expertise, high intelligence, the capability to communicate with coworkers, and an appropriate background of reliable and honest work patterns. The main difficulty in the selective process lies in the area of their emotional maturity, their capacity to evaluate co-workers in depth, the presence of adequate, "paranoid" features—non-naïve critical evaluation and "narcissistic" features—the ability to stand up to criticism and unavoidable institutional aggression. The situation is much more complex in the case of selecting political leadership. Candidates with severely paranoid and narcissistic features and even antisocial behavior may be well aware of the need to present themselves as open and friendly, attentive to others' wishes and needs, and disguise their resentful selfishness and self-absorption, and their true thinking, if the moment "is not right." Madeline Albright (2018) has described the erroneous impression Hitler conveyed in early interviews, and her own experience with Chavez (Venezuela's former president) and other political leaders that did not reveal their true personality. It is regarding newly emerging, radical movements that the danger of their so well fitting malignant narcissistic leadership be ignored—with unfortunate consequences. It is obvious that there are historical moments in which powerful social forces may operate in the direction of splitting off of social subgroups, including the unavoidable disorganizing effects of economic crises and political chaos.

Jacques Semelin (2007) recommends international action and the responsibility of the social sciences. He believes that, in the international field, individual nations as well as the United Nations have to adopt ethical responsibility, including the responsibility to prevent social crises that are manmade and put populations in danger. The United Nations should react in the face of situations where the protection of human beings impresses the necessity of resorting to appropriate, including coercive, measures, accepting the responsibility to intervene, facilitating receiving military rescue intervention, providing assistance to resumption of reconstruction, and reconciliation. In terms of the responsibility of the social sciences, he believes that the social researcher has at least to take on the responsibility to make known our accumulating knowledge of the causes of social crisis and particularly genocide. The study of genocide is an essential, urgent need for the field of the social sciences, and that includes psychoanalysis. Psychoanalysis can contribute with the understanding of the psychology of large group regression, the psychology of the syndrome of malignant narcissism, and more generally, the interaction between leadership pathology and group regression. Psychoanalytic contributions to the understanding of optimal leadership in social institutions may be a helpful contribution to the evaluation of political leaders as well.

Here the contribution of the distinguished historian Timothy Snyder (2017) is relevant (*On Tyranny: Twenty Lessons From the Twentieth Century*). His 20 lessons include the call to institutions to distrust one-party states and be wary of power militias. We must remember professional ethics, believe in truth, investigate, and listen for dangerous words. He explains the importance of establishing a private life, contributing to good causes, learning from peers of other countries. He affirms that it is important to be calm when the unthinkable arrives, be a patriot, and be as courageous as one can. He thus outlines a profile of individual courage, responsibility, independence of thinking, and public action. I think these are eminently reasonable and, in fact, essential qualities that permit the individual to stand up to the dangerous imprisonment in regressive group formations and confront dishonest, corrupting, and corrupted leadership. In the political arena, malignant narcissistic leadership should not be exposed with diagnostic psychiatrist labels but by pointing to their public, cohesively pathological, characteristic behavior. From a psychoanalytic perspective, the development of a strong personal identity, with its related capacity to evaluate oneself and others in depth, to respect the right for privacy and individual boundaries as well as boundaries for the couple in love and for the family are important contributions to the achievement of the individual stance that is described by Timothy Snyder, and so are the psychoanalytic contributions to our understanding of the psychology of small and large regressed groups and their ideological consequences. And the understanding of dangerous personality formations in social leaders may help the prevention of the toxic combination of regressed groups and malignant leaders.

References

Albright M: Fascism: A Warning. New York, Harper Collins, 2018

Bao-Lord B: Legacies: A Chinese Mosaic. New York, Fawcett Columbine, 1990

Bion W: Experiences in Groups. London, Tavistock, 1961

Canetti E: Masse und Macht. Frankfurt am Main, Germany, Fischer Taschen-
buch Verlag, 1960

Freud S: Group psychology and the analysis of the ego (1921), in The Standard
Edition of the Complete Psychological Works of Sigmund Freud, Vol 18.
Translated and edited by Strachey J. London, Hogarth, 1949, pp 63–143

Jacques E: A General Theory of Bureaucracy. New York Halsted, 1976

Kernberg O: Severe Personality Disorders: Psychotherapeutic Strategies. New
Haven, CT, Yale University Press, 1984

Kernberg O: Ideology, Conflict, and Leadership in Groups and Organizations.
New Haven, CT, Yale University Press, 1998

Kernberg O: Sanctioned social violence: a psychoanalytic view. Int J Psychoanal
84:953–968, 2003

Kernberg O: Treatment of Severe Personality Disorders: Resolution of Aggression and Recovery of Eroticism. Washington, DC, American Psychiatric Association Publishing, 2018

Klein M: Notes on some schizoid mechanisms. Int J Psychoanal 27:99–110, 1946

Moscovici S: L'Age des Folles. Paris, Libraire Arthèma Fayard, 1981

Semelin J: Purify and Destroy: The Political Uses of Massacre and Genocide.
New York, Columbia University Press, 2007

Snyder T: On Tyranny: Twenty Lessons From the Twentieth Century. New York,
Tim Duggan Books, 2017

Turquet P: Threats to identity in the large group, in The Large Group: Dynamics
and Therapy. Edited by Kreeger L. London, Karnac, 1975

Volkan V: Blind Trust. Charlottesville, VA, Pitchstone, 2004

CHAPTER 12

Challenges for the Future of Psychoanalysis

Present-Day Challenges

I believe there exists a general consensus in the psychoanalytic community that psychoanalysis is going through a very difficult time, which many believe to be a true crisis. Psychoanalysis has had a well-established place in the development of Western culture during the 20th century, and its cultural influences extend to the present. The psychoanalytic concern with fundamental issues in psychology, particularly the influence of unconscious processes on psychological functioning, has promoted major scientific progress in the psychological sciences.

As a mental health profession psychoanalysis represents major organizations in Europe, North and South America, Asia, South Africa, and Australia. However, although its contribution to culture and to the humanities has been universally recognized, in recent years the scientific status of psychoanalysis has been questioned, and psychoanalytic orga-

Published in the *American Journal of Psychoanalysis* 81(3):281–300, 2021. Copyright © 2021 Association for the Advancement of Psychoanalysis. Reprinted with permission.

nizations have faced a diminished level of interest from the broader mental health community and the intellectual, academic, and scientific world at large. External challenges to psychoanalysis have been matched by internal conflicts affecting the psychoanalytic community. As a profession, psychoanalysis is experiencing a declining prestige in its surrounding social and cultural environment. Questions have been raised about its effectiveness, the lack of research on its effectiveness, and serious competition has evolved with the availability of alternative treatments, such as psychopharmacological treatment and cognitive-behavioral approaches to psychotherapy.

The division of the psychoanalytic field into "classical" psychoanalysis, which is taught in specialized institutes, and psychoanalytic psychotherapy, which consists of a widely developed field of diversified psychotherapies, presents a confusing image to the outside world. The objective scientific contributions of psychoanalysis are virtually paralyzed by the lack of systematic training and dedication to research. The internal controversies about alternative new approaches to psychoanalytic theory and practice have not been studied scientifically, nor has any legitimate scientific comparative analysis been made on psychoanalysis versus other approaches. Therefore, support for any one approach over another has been based primarily on ideological commitments rather than on objective comparison of their effectiveness.

Many psychoanalytic societies and institutes face problems due to controversial aspects of the training analyst system. The traditional organization of psychoanalytic education has led to the development of an elite corps of training analysts, who have exerted a dysfunctional and authoritarian power over how educational training programs and psychoanalytic societies at large are run. Conflict within the psychoanalytic training community have caused two major problems: first, there has been no agreement on the definition of psychoanalytic competence, nor the educational and practical standards that training institutes must provide to ensure that candidates meet this level of competence; and second, the adverse effects that these conflicts have had on candidates, educators, and the certification process. Furthermore, there has been a remarkable resistance to establishing a clear definition of professional competence, and standards to achieve it, which has gravely affected professional education and the reputation of psychoanalysis as an important field of study.

In recent years, a polarity has arisen in our community as to how we resolve these issues. One viewpoint is that our field of study should be seen as a scientific enterprise, subject to the usual standards of scientific exploration and empirical research, with clear methodologies and assessment criteria. The opposite point of view sees our field of study in humanistic terms that cannot be subjected to the usual rules and measurements of objective science—it is an enterprise that deals with the unique subjective, creative, and rich exploratory experiences of individuals and the particularities of the analytic couple/dyad.

Practically, this dichotomy has found expression in the repeated concern over the "identity" of the psychoanalyst and the extent to which this identity reflects an identity appropriate to any professional who adheres to the values of his particular profession while carrying out its associated tasks. This idea contrasts with the assumption that psychoanalysis is unique because it explores the dynamic unconscious, which requires a particular empathy and commitment to the spiritual values of individual mental functioning that transcends the limited, strictly "technical" identification with the various aspects of professional competence.

Efforts to reduce the authoritarian nature of psychoanalytic education have been carried out in various parts of the world. There have been significant efforts at innovating educational processes by creating objective criteria for choosing candidates and providing more instruction by non-training analysts, many of whom have educational expertise without having achieved training analyst status (Zagermann 2017). These developments, however, have shed a light on the psychoanalytic community's "secret" doubt about the quality of its own educational system and the competence level of its graduates because there have been few standards for either and no method of assessing their effectiveness. This has meant that only a few graduates are eligible or selected to become training analysts.

The implication, of course, is that if the criteria for psychoanalytic competence were clear, transparent, objective, and measurable and if psychoanalytic education were geared to produce professionals that fulfilled the criteria, then every graduate would qualify as a training analyst. In fact, optimal training would produce *only* training analysts, as it does in other medical specialties, where it is understood that once an appropriate level of competence is achieved, there is a corresponding competence to carry out clinical, research, and educational functions. Efforts to innovate psychoanalytic education by implementing objective criteria for education, assessment, and certification are often thwarted by the prevailing ideological assumption that psychoanalysis is not a science. Because this unspecified nature of the profession has been preserved, its evaluation has often been relegated to the quality of the psychoanalyst—specifically, to his or her unique ability to attune to manifestations of the unconscious. Thus, the conflict between the psychoanalyst as either scientist or humanist protects the established elites in the profession from using objective processes to select training analysts to carry out the educational functions of their institutes (Kernberg 2016).

A complicating factor, which I would suggest has upended the central focus on establishing standards, lies in how psychoanalysis is practiced in different countries. French psychoanalysts are trained with three sessions a week, British psychoanalysts with five sessions a week, and the majority of psychoanalytic institutes in Europe and North America with four sessions a week. Here again, tradition, rather than empirical findings, has determined subjective convictions of validity, and the highest frequency institutes have adopted a somewhat derogatory attitude toward the lower frequency institutes, often categorizing their practice as "not real psychoanalysis."

Instead of concern about having universal standards for developing and certifying professional competence, the struggle has devolved into a political battle for institutional dominance based on the recommended frequency of sessions. Obviously, research on the effectiveness of training that looks at similar methods with different numbers of sessions would provide valuable information, but the absence of agreed upon standards precludes undertaking any effective empirical studies.

It seems reasonable to assume that a minimum of three sessions per week should be required in the practice of classical psychoanalysis. Severely narcissistic personality structures would probably benefit from having four or even five sessions per week, given their difficulty with establishing deep human connection and engagement. This is a decision to be made on an individual basis. However, there are other issues that impede the creation of standards, and these include less traditional modes of treatment, some of which work better for certain populations. So, we will now shift our focus to them.

Modified Psychoanalytic Psychotherapies

Modified psychoanalytic psychotherapies, with sessions once or twice weekly, have been studied scientifically and are effective in treating personality disorders that do not respond well to standard psychoanalytic treatment (Bateman et al. 2016; Caligor et al. 2018; Luyten et al. 2015; Rudolf 2019; Yeomans et al. 2015). Their success has raised questions about how useful these techniques might be with a broader range of patients. Empirical research has been conducted on transference-focused psychotherapy (TFP), mentalization-based psychotherapy (MBT), and German depth psychology-oriented psychotherapy (TPOP). All of these have manualized descriptions of their technical approaches and the methodologies used to evaluate their effectiveness. I believe this reflects an unexpected and truly revolutionary confirmation that psychoanalytic instruments are effective as a general treatment for psychological illness. Yet, most psychoanalytic institutes have been strongly opposed to including modified analytic procedures in their educational programs despite independent research that supports the effectiveness of these approaches.

This elitist stance perpetuates the educational crises in our profession through self-induced isolation, rejection, and neglect of research which has alienated academic and university mental health programs from psychoanalysis. The response by psychoanalysis has been to voice concern about the authoritarianism of the training analyst system and to debate frequency of treatment without empirical investigation. Neglected are defining criteria for professional competence, studying the place of comparative research to assess treatment effectiveness and what are the effective elements operating in psychoanalytic psychotherapies as well as in standard psychoanalysis. What is to be done?

Potential Solutions

SPECIFIC THEORETICAL CHALLENGES

To begin, I shall explore our tasks at the level of psychoanalytic theory and its applications and our psychoanalytic technique and its applications. This is the body of our science, and the first task, I believe, is to bring theory and technique up to date with our present knowledge and experience and to the level at which research for future development is indicated and possibly urgent.

Regarding theory, psychoanalytic object relations theory has gradually influenced and transformed almost all contemporary psychoanalytic theory and practice: perceiving the organization, development, behavior manifestations, and psychopathology that psychoanalysis has explored from the viewpoint of the vicissitudes of unconscious conflicts and their derived psychopathological structures.

Here, psychoanalysis has looked to the neighboring field of neurobiology to examine the neurobiological determinants of activation of unconscious processes, the nature of drives as original motivational systems, and the defenses built against them. Along with this, we have encountered two major areas that require integration into psychoanalytic thinking: contemporary neurobiological affect theory and the expanded view of unconscious cognitive processes. There are good reasons to consider inborn affect systems, operating as temperamental dispositions from birth on and providing the immediate motivational drive to engage in relations with significant others—primarily mother (Panksepp and Biven 2012; Solms 2015).

This basic development in neurobiological understanding is relevant to the psychoanalytic theory of drives. Should drive theory be replaced by affect theory? Or should we ask how these two theoretical frames relate from the standpoint of contemporary findings in both fields?

The discovery of the enormous importance of unconscious procedural memory functions that complement and extend fundamentally the concept of the unconscious dynamic raises the question how all these modalities of unconscious developments relate to the psychoanalytic concept of the dynamic unconscious? How does the evidence for originally conscious affective processes in the infant relate to the assumption of the originally unconscious nature of the dynamic unconscious?

These are some fundamental questions that require expanding psychoanalytic inquiry into the interrelationship between neurobiological and psychodynamic phenomena, structures, and development. Our present-day knowledge of the neurobiological aspects of genetic predisposition to major depressive illness requires the expansion of our psychodynamic theories of depression with the consideration of the neurobiological basis of the pathology of depressive affect. Similarly, other psychic symptoms that we now understand better in terms of their neurobiological disposition, such as anxiety reactions, dissociative phenomena, and the capacity for assessing emotionally significant others, are areas that concern us. Neurocognitive structures, affect systems, memory development, and inborn adaptive potentials should inform and enrich important psychoanalytic assumptions. How do neurobiological predispositions interact with the effects of object relations from birth on? Clearly, psychoanalysis must do a better job of incorporating neurobiological findings that have relevance for both psychoanalytic theory and its practice.

At the same time, contemporary psychoanalytic object relations theory has stressed that the earliest self-representations are dyadic in nature and develop in interaction with the representations of significant others, in the context of a dominant affect state that links self and object. We see that these earliest psychological developments are linked to many interpersonal relationships: couples, families, groups, and societies. Object relations can reveal important unconscious motivations that express themselves interpersonally, ideologically, politically, and socially.

Freud (1921/1949) had already opened up this field with his contributions to the study of group psychology, and our knowledge has advanced significantly with the work of psychoanalytically inspired sociologists (Moscovici 1981) and politically interested psychoanalysts (Volkan 2004).

Psychoanalysis and sociology have much to offer each other. It is important for sociologists to understand the impact of psychoanalytic advances on society as a whole. For example, how unconscious psychoanalytic processes can motivate group regression and the self-destructive behaviors that threaten the equilibrium of society, so evident in the 20th century and those we are witnessing today. Psychoanalysts must also familiarize themselves with contemporary sociological, organizational, and historical studies to understand social factors that have psychological impacts on individuals and society. Ultimately, it may be necessary to create psychoanalytic subspecialties that have important social and political implications.

CHALLENGES OF PSYCHOANALYTIC TECHNIQUE

The fields of neurobiology and sociology have made incredible advances in the study of individual and group behavior, but these are largely underexploited in terms of psychoanalytic inquiry. Psychoanalytic institutions have been indifferent, if not hostile, to expanding their knowledge base to include other disciplines in their training or research programs, or in making essential psychoanalytic contributions to society.

Alternative psychoanalytic techniques within competing contemporary psychoanalytic schools have enriched our practice with many helpful therapeutic interventions, such as those found in many psychoanalytically based contemporary therapies. These include contemporary ego psychology, contemporary Kleinian psychology, Neo-Bionian psychology, contemporary relational psychoanalysis, and contemporary French psychoanalysis (with significant influences from Lacanian thinking) (Kernberg 2018). What seems most important here is not competing over alternative ways of applying standard psychoanalytic technique but how to organize them into an integrated concept of psychoanalytic technique that then permits developing overall modifications or modifications to specific components of psychoanalytic technique. Such a reworking would help consolidate those aspects that have proven to be particularly effective in the treatment of certain groups of patients.

I cannot overstate the importance of having foundational reference points for psychoanalytic technique that integrate the common components—neutrality, interpretation, dream analysis, transference, countertransference, holding, acting out, termination, etc.—under the shared rubric of the psychology and the psychopathology of the dynamic unconscious. It is astonishing that there isn't a single text which recognizes and teaches traditional or classic psychoanalytic technique as an integrated set of overarching principles from which various schools may have developed alternative modifications. Without such a work, in my own experience, instruction about technique has been practically chaotic in terms of sequences of courses on the various components of the technique and doesn't give psychoanalytic candidates a way to internalize a basic orientation to the field. Interpretation, transference analysis, character analysis, acting out, negative therapeutic reaction, dream analysis, termination, containment and holding, and therapeutic alliance tend to be taught as relatively independent subjects. In addition, some analysts from the "humanistic" segment favor extreme "anti-technical" positions that support methods based on highly individual preferences, and many personally achieved fame doing so.

COMPREHENSIVE INTEGRATED BODY OF PSYCHOANALYTIC TECHNIQUES

We have attempted to modify psychoanalytic technique quite successfully, I believe, in the construction of TFP as a modified psychoanalytic technique used to treat severe personality disorders (Yeomans et al. 2015). We have distinguished four basic psychoanalytic techniques—interpretation, transference analysis, technical neutrality, and countertransference utilization, described their essential mutual relationships, and specified how each technique can be modified for TFP. Our effort demonstrates the possibility of defining the fundamental elements of psychoanalytic technique that can be applied equally well to traditional psychoanalysis and, with slight modification, to psychoanalytic psychotherapies.

The point is that a clear conceptualization of psychoanalytic technique would permit its expanded application, and this standardization might then better enable comparative studies of different psychotherapies. We could automatically study the extent to which, for example, the use of the couch contrasts with face-to-face interventions, or the predominant use of free associations contrasts with behavioral analysis in relation to transference developments in their application to different types of patients. This specific application of a combination of psychoanalytic interventions stands in stark contrast to the "diluted" approach practiced today by traditionally trained analysts who have no specific training in psychoanalytic psychotherapy. Some practitioners assume that seeing patients in a sitting up, face-to-face position rather than lying on the couch and using selective psychoanalytic techniques as they see fit constitutes a form of psychoanalytic psychotherapy. There is empirical evidence that truly manualized forms of psychotherapy designed for specific psychopathologies are more effective than vague, unstructured psychoanalytic or psychodynamic psychotherapies.

Psychoanalytic institutes that incorporate comprehensive, specific, and integrated techniques in their training could help the psychoanalytic clinician develop expertise in treating patients from a broad spectrum of functioning, including those with severely regressed personality disorders for whom psychoanalysis is usually contraindicated, thereby improving the social relevance of psychoanalysis and possibly restoring its prestige as a viable treatment option.

Psychoanalytic candidates would learn specific treatments like MBT, TFP, TPOP, or supportive psychotherapy based on psychoanalytic principles. They would also learn to conduct psychoanalytic treatment for groups, families, and couples (a major clinical challenge these days). There is a wealth of expertise dispersed across these fields, but they are completely disconnected from the psychoanalytic training community, preventing research about the therapeutic moderators and mediators of the overall effectiveness of various psychoanalytic treatments.

THE PLACE OF RESEARCH, PHILOSOPHY, AND ART

If there is going to be integrated research to investigate and develop integrated applied psychoanalytic theories and techniques, institutes will need to require specialized faculty who are experts on the relationships between psychoanalysis and their specific fields. Diversifying faculty will enrich both the psychoanalytic faculty and, by implication, the institutional interest in developing a broader knowledge base. At the same time, a diverse faculty should necessitate a robust research department to investigate current trends in corresponding fields and to identify methodologies for research projects emanating from within the institute.

Significant empirical research has already been carried out in the field of psychoanalytic psychotherapies (for example, American Psychological Association 2013; Kernberg 2015; Wallerstein 2014), meaning that psychoanalysis already has access to expert research designers and instrument developers, though more will be needed. This focus on scientific development and research in relation to other sciences emphasizes the scientific aspects of psychoanalysis

At the same time, psychoanalysis must always stay alert to the existential, intersubjective, philosophical, and humanistic aspects of the study of the unconscious in individual psychoanalysis (for example, Akhtar 2010; Civitarese 2018; Weigert 1964).

It must maintain openness to the creative aspect of the unconscious, to creativity in the areas of art, religion, and philosophy, which are involved in what psychoanalytic treatment may foster in the individual psychoanalytic experience of patients with relatively less severe illness who have clear indication for standard psychoanalysis.

Persons without any particular therapeutic reasons may be interested in undergoing psychoanalysis to become better acquainted with the unconscious aspects of their minds, to deepen the richness of their personal experience, or to understand internal conflicts that may affect their creativity. Psychoanalysis has important existential implications for patients and analysts within all psychoanalytic orientations who are focused on these goals, and it represents an ideological concern for psychoanalysts who are mostly dedicated to the standard psychoanalytic treatment of better functioning patients. It is this group of analysts, who are concerned that scientific research means a superficialization and mechanization of psychoanalysis, who need to be reassured of the commitment to this dimension of psychoanalysis that indeed transcends the practical requirement for treatment of mental illness that society expects from psychoanalysis. In other words, we must preserve the humanistic aspect of the psychoanalytic "movement." The scientific and existential aspects of psychoanalysis are not in conflict: it is the growing authoritarianism in psychoanalytic institutes that continues to motivate this conflictual split. Especially since existential and philosophical questions come up in the treatment of patients who are having more serious problems as well.

PSYCHOANALYSIS AND ACADEMIA

Everything I've said to this point about the need to both acquire existing knowledge and develop new knowledge underscores the importance of integrating psychoanalytic education and research with academia. The purpose would be to maintain a psychoanalytic presence and investigative spirit throughout the university and acquire expertise in the related subjects that may be relevant for psychoanalytic theory and technique. It would also encourage the development of interdisciplinary research, and it would provide the live, daily interchange between developments in university settings and psychoanalytic institutions that may foster interest, development of knowledge, and particularly the development of relevant research programs. How can we achieve this?

I am proposing two major approaches to resolve the alienation of organized psychoanalysis from the university. First, as mentioned, all candidates in training should be exposed to the various specialty areas of psychoanalytic therapy and technique; this should stimulate parallel interest in training and faculty status in these new specialties at universities. In other words, psychoanalytic candidates, as well as their teachers, should attempt to achieve faculty status, respectively, in departments of psychiatry, clinical psychology, social work, the arts, religion, philosophy, political science, administrative leadership, and even economics and mathematics. The purpose would be to maintain a psychoanalytic presence and investigative spirit throughout the university and acquire expertise in the related subjects that may be relevant for psychoanalytic theory and technique. It would also encourage the development of interdisciplinary research. This would provide the live, daily interchange between developments in university settings and psychoanalytic institutions that may foster interest, development of knowledge, and particularly the development of relevant research programs. This collaborative spirit isn't new. In the last century, especially in Germany and the United States, most psychoanalysts have had links with university departments of psychiatry or clinical psychology. Having psychoanalysts in the student body and/or on the faculty of various university departments such as neuroscience, sociology, political science, etc., would offer extraordinary opportunities for the cross-fertilization of ideas.

The second aspect is more subtle, complex, and dependent on the very different local situations. In various countries there could be an ongoing, concerted effort of psychoanalytic institutions to establish and maintain contact between the leadership of psychoanalytic institutions and university faculty, and to establish and maintain collegial relationships at the top administrative levels of the respective institutions, particularly department chairs. This could be done, for example, by inviting leading neurological scientists to attend or possibly to speak at symposia on depressive psychopathology organized by psychoanalytic societies or by inviting political science professors to participate in a conference on the psychoanalytic aspects of social regression to violence. This would enrich psychoanalytic programs as well as their relationship with universities.

It would be naive not to recognize the present biases and prejudices about psychoanalysis within university settings that include, unfortunately, well justified resentment because of past times, when the psychoanalytic dominance of some departments of psychiatry or clinical psychology evinced a regrettable lack of psychoanalytic interest or even demonstrated contempt regarding the biological aspect of psychiatric illness and treatment. I believe that only such an ongoing, concerted effort will be helpful to organically integrate psychoanalysis with academia.

Questions as to whether psychoanalytic institutes should remain completely independent or partially included in a university system should be answered pragmatically, based on many factors, not the least of which are the different sociocultural traditions and the academic standing of the university. The many different psychoanalytic theories and clinical approaches and the very complexity of educating candidates would seem to justify maintaining relatively independent psychoanalytic institutions. This is particularly so in countries with large, diversified specializations, especially in the natural and humanistic sciences. In a smaller city, it might be easier to achieve integration, and there may be advantages to being part of a large university system.

PSYCHOANALYTIC CENTERS

Regardless of where they are located, psychoanalytic institutions or "centers" should be integrated organizations that include several components. First, there would ideally be a research department concentrating on research design, collecting and sharing relevant research information from elsewhere, fostering intra- and interdepartmental research and providing ongoing support and quality control. Second, there would be an educational training department that organizes, develops, and integrates relevant psychoanalytic psychotherapies within standard psychoanalytic training. This could specializations, such as group therapy or couples therapy, but basic psychoanalytic training would form the foundation of each specialty. Third, there would be a department of professional development, responsible for membership retention within the psychoanalytic community. This could be organized as a psychoanalytic society with specialized subgroups. The department would be responsible for developing specific postgraduate educational programs, conferences, and meetings and for corresponding to the needs of psychoanalysts working in all specialties. Fourth, there would be a department of community relations, which would be responsible for establishing and maintaining relationships between the institution and its academic, cultural, and political cohorts. This department would also coordinate the engagement of the psychoanalytic leadership with academic or community leadership in related areas of interest. The concept of a "psychoanalytic center" works well as an umbrella organization for these four departments: research, education, professional development, and community relations. An executive committee representing these various areas would be responsible for overall governance of the institution, and the leaders of each segment could preside over the internal organization appropriate to the nature of their specific tasks. Organizations of this type are already developing within the United States. Their generalization may help to end old conflicts between psychoanalytic institutes and psychoanalytic societies that have prevailed internationally.

STANDARDS FOR CERTIFICATION

How psychoanalytic education has been organized is at the very center of the debates causing these longstanding battles, so it should be the first area of focus. As mentioned, its number one priority is to define psychoanalytic competence. This means developing standards for training and creating a certification process that ensures that each candidate who successfully completes a program has the necessary training, skills, and ability to provide specific treatments for mental illness. The title of psychoanalyst, therefore, would refer only to those mental health professionals who have been fully and reliably trained in all clinical therapeutic modalities based on psychoanalytic theory and technique and who are authorized to treat patients and psychoanalytic candidates. This certification would imply competence in standard psychoanalysis, TFP, MBT, etc., and confirm that the graduate analyst has the broad and diversified clinical skills needed to carry out one or several of these psychoanalytically based clinical applications.

Such certification is not only possible but essential. TFP and other psychoanalytic psychotherapies, such as TPOP, provide clear and succinct definitions of competence, which can also be applied to psycho-analytic technique at psychoanalytic institutes. The current training analyst system could be abolished.

A NEW CURRICULUM

The new curriculum could include relevant developments in boundary fields, and experts in those fields could become part of the teaching faculty. As mentioned, such a program would generate excitement and stimulate creative developments in psychoanalytic institutes. So much of psychoanalytic theory is based on a historical review from the beginning of Freud's work to this time, without emphasizing current theory. Updated psychoanalytic concepts on development, psychological structure, and psychopathology may be synthesized, and presently controversial concepts spelled out within a 4-year program. Psychoanalytic experience should occur alongside education, leaving the candidate and certified psychoanalyst to decide on the arrangements of treatment. When the question of session frequency emerges, we should be clear that while it may be preferable to have higher frequency of contact between therapist and patient, we have no scientific evidence showing significantly different effects from psychoanalysis at five, four, or three sessions per week. Different psychoanalytic centers have different ways of approaching this issue, and the psychoanalytic community has debated its importance for over 50 years but has never studied it empirically. Having a clearer definition of the effectiveness of treatment measures could possibly help resolve the issue. The particular customs may continue, but clearly, authentic research about the effectiveness of treatment is needed.

Simultaneous training in the treatment of both well-functioning individuals and those with more serious personality disorders could be very useful. It would improve the clinical experience, intensify the awareness and management of psychoanalytic instruments, and accelerate intensive training while at the same time providing sufficient patients to all candidates. It could also give candidates access to much-needed income during their training.

Professionals in other disciplines interested in psychoanalytic theory and its applications without the inclination to become therapists might become associate members of a psychoanalytic center. They could focus on a particular specialization in the various departments of research, professional development, and community relations, and would be granted full membership rights. Their participation in any one of these four areas would be beneficial. They could inspire the development of interesting interdisciplinary research projects; teach a broader curriculum to psychoanalytic candidates; participate in and encourage others to attend psychoanalytic symposia; and help introduce psychoanalysis as a field and the psychoanalytic center as a resource to a wider audience. These activities would greatly contribute to the seriously neglected objective of integrating peripheral functions into psychoanalysis.

EVALUATING COMPETENCE

Curricular content should be based on an agreed-upon definition of psychoanalytic competence and whatever knowledge and experience is required for candidates to meet that definition and become certified as analysts. Körner (2002) and Tuckett (2005) have made important advances regarding the criteria of psychoanalytic competence. Körner suggests evaluating psychoanalytic competence based on three criteria: knowledge, technical capacity, and analytic attitude. We already have educational benchmarks and clinical standards by which to evaluate a candidate's proficiency in each of these areas in the current psychoanalytic certifying examination. Tuckett has also proposed three major features of psychoanalytic competence. First is the capacity to carefully describe and assess all available data that the analyst has obtained in the analytic session. Second is the ability to formulate a psychoanalytic hypothesis that brings together the underlying dynamics and observed facts that will constitute the main source for interpretive intervention. And third is the skill to find appropriate interpretive interventions that satisfactorily convey these dynamic understandings in the therapeutic interaction. Again, these reflect general criteria that have to be elaborated into their constituents, but they illustrate the extent to which the definition of psychoanalytic competence and its realistic evaluation is perfectly feasible.

What do we mean by psychoanalytic "attitude" and, in a more general sense, psychoanalytic "identity," and how do we evaluate this? Evaluating a candidate's competence in psychoanalytic technique is becoming recognized as somewhat feasible in terms of our present-day experience, but is there something unique about the "identity" of the analyst that cannot be measured, except intuitively when interacting with any particular candidate? Meetings and conferences have been dedicated to this question for years, and the two main attitudinal requirements of an analyst seem to be 1) the willingness and capacity to listen carefully, being entirely open and attuned to everything being communicated by the patient, consciously and unconsciously, while being equally attuned to his own internal reactions to these communications; and 2) the ability to tolerate the uncertainty, of "not knowing" as a precondition for letting the unexpected emerge in one's understanding of self and the other in any analytic interaction. It points, on the one hand, to the establishment and observation of free association as a basic task expected from the patient, and an openness to the variety of countertransference developments that occur on an ongoing basis in the context of each therapeutic interaction. Recent literature, particularly under the influence of the Neo-Bionian School, has focused on the analyst's "reverie," a slightly bewildering concept that Fred Busch (2019) explores in his book, *The Analyst's Reverie: Exploration in Bion's Enigmatic Concept*. Busch concludes that *reverie* or *daydreaming* can help clarify the therapist's reaction to the material that surfaces when interacting with the patient.

The achievement of professional competence requires extensive, highly specialized theoretical education and many long hours of experiential training in clinical practice, and these basic requirements must be clearly spelled out, provided in a reasonable sequence, and integrated into a comprehensive curriculum of classical psychoanalytic theory and technique. Evaluation methods, by subject matter and class year, should support and complement a carefully tended path to becoming a highly competent professional.

REQUIRED PERSONAL PSYCHOANALYSIS

Each candidate's personal psychoanalysis would develop completely independently from other aspects of their psychoanalytic training, although personal psychoanalysis should be required of all candidates who wish to become certified. It seems reasonable that the psychoanalytic institution be informed of candidates' being in the process or having carried out such an experience. In the end, a candidate's willingness and ability to explore his own dynamic unconscious through deep experiences and conflicts can only be evaluated by how well he is able to capture corresponding transference experiences in the treatment of patients. In short, a candidate really needs to undergo his own psychoanalysis before attempting to treat someone else.

The supervisor would have a fundamental role in psychoanalytic education. A supervising body should arrange the training experiences so that supervisors are able to gain adequate knowledge of a trainee's capabilities, difficulties, and problems and the extent to which they can be resolved as part of their educational experience. It would seem fundamental that supervisors communicate openly with each other and with the candidate as well. Group supervision is an excellent way to give candidates a broader view of human conflicts, therapeutic processes, and exposure to their colleagues' wider experience. This will also support shared group learning processes within the institution.

LEADERSHIP

Faculty from a department with a particular specialty should select leaders for their component of the psychoanalytic center. Of course, the direction of a center within a university will be influenced by its administrative structure, and an autonomous center might be administered differently. Nonetheless, selecting its leadership from the entire faculty of the center would assure objectivity and encourage organizational feedback about problems with its administrative structure. Allowing the entire faculty to choose leaders from within its ranks differs from the current system where training analysts select the leadership of psychoanalytic institutes. Eliminating the training analyst system altogether should have a healthy influence on the administrative structure. But, first, as mentioned, many important goals will have to be met: defining psychoanalytic competence; creating educational standards and a clear, objective, and transparent certification process; along with national and international work of the psychoanalytic community to ensure a consistent definition of competence in all clinical psychoanalysts.

PROFESSIONAL IDENTITY

I believe that professional identity derives from the interest, commitment, effectiveness, and gratification in carrying out a specific profession, and the identity of the psychoanalyst should come from the gratification of carrying out the psychoanalytic tasks. The fear that psychoanalytic psychotherapy would "dilute" the work and identity of the psychoanalyst comes from an idealized version of the profession and, at a deeper level, a fear that the original psychoanalytic enterprise won't survive. This shouldn't concern psychoanalysts trained to provide standard psychoanalysis and specialized psychoanalytic psychotherapies. On the contrary, the increased effectiveness of therapeutic intervention from widening one's knowledge base and skills should be a source of gratification and pride, as should the sense of making an authentic contribution to mental health in the community. Specialization that deepens a particular aspect of the psychoanalytic endeavor may even powerfully reinforce one's identity. Experts who work with specific types of clients may wish to expand their approach to serve others, as Eve Caligor did when she extended TFP to the entire field of personality disorders (Caligor et al. 2018). Psychoanalysts interested in standard psychoanalytic technique, still the main focus of psychoanalytic institutes, could form innovative study groups, create research projects, and make tremendous intellectual contributions that a psychoanalytic center would fundamentally support and promote.

SPECIALIZATION

I have not even touched upon specialization. One area of great importance is child and adolescent psychoanalysis, which could be its own division within the department of education. A highly relevant and fundamental aspect of psychoanalytic theory and technique is the study of early development, particularly the relationship between neurobiological predispositions and psychological functioning and the nature of early psychosocial, especially familiar influences on personality development (Ackerman 2010). Experts from within this specialized division of child and adolescent psychoanalysis could reach out to professionals in many other fields and collaborate on projects of interest to both. There are many experts to tap in fields as disparate as neuroscience, biology, sociology, general psychology, education, or more closely related fields like mother–infant relations. These experts and, more generally, non-psychoanalytic professionals could join the center as associate members to help us broaden our knowledge base and complement many fundamental components of the total psychoanalytic enterprise.

Another important area of psychoanalytic contribution to the community as well as a boundary to the social sciences is the psychoanalytic study of organizational structure and conflict, One example comes from a collaboration in which psychoanalyst experts consulted with industries in Germany, Great Britain, and the United States and produced a psychoanalytic study of organizational structure and conflict (Sievers 2009).

These are just a few examples of what psychoanalysis has to offer the world, but also, what it has to learn. Interdisciplinary work is the springboard for learning but also for innovation and authentic mutual enrichment that every science typically experiences at its boundaries.

References

Ackerman S: Is infant research useful in clinical work with adults? J Am Psychoanal Assoc 58:1201–1211, 2010

Akhtar S: Happiness: origins, forms and technical relevance. Am J Psychoanal 70(3):219–244, 2010

American Psychological Association: Recognition of psychotherapy effectiveness. Psychotherapy 50:102–109, 2013

Bateman A, Fonagy P: Mentalization-Based Treatment for Borderline Personality Disorder: A Practical Guide, 2nd Edition. New York, Oxford University Press, 2016

Busch F: The Analyst's Reverie: Exploration in Bion's Enigmatic Concept. London, Routledge, 2019

Caligor E, Kernberg OF, Clarkin JF, Yeomans FE: Psychodynamic Therapy for Personality Pathology. Washington, DC, American Psychiatric Association Publishing, 2018

Civitarese G: Sublime Subjects: Aesthetic Experience and Intersubjectivity in Psychoanalysis. Abingdon, NY, Routledge, 2018

Freud S: Group psychology and the analysis of the ego (1921), in The Standard Edition of the Complete Psychological Works of Sigmund Freud, Vol 18. Translated and edited by Strachey J. London, Hogarth, 1949, pp 65–144

Kernberg OF: Resistances and progress in developing a research framework in psychoanalytic institutes. Psychoanal Inq 35(suppl):98–114, 2015

Kernberg OF: Psychoanalytic Education at the Crossroads. London, Routledge, 2016

Kernberg OF: Resolution of Aggression and Recovery of Eroticism: Treatment of Severe Personality Disorders. Washington, DC, American Psychiatric Association Publishing, 2018

Körner J: The didactics of psychoanalytic education. Int J Psychoanal 83:1395–1405, 2002

Luyten P, Mayes L, Fonagy P, et al: Handbook for Psychodynamic Approaches to Psychopathology. New York, Guilford, 2015

Moscovici S: L'Age des Foules. Paris, Arthème Feyard, 1981

Panksepp J, Biven L: The Archaeology of the Mind. New York, Norton, 2012

Rudolf G: Psychodynamisch Denken: Tiefenpsychologisch Handeln. Stuttgart, Germany, Schattauer, 2019

Sievers B (ed): Psychoanalytic Studies of Organizations: Contributions From the International Society for the Psychoanalytic Study of Organizations (ISPSO). New York, Routledge, 2009

Solms M: The Feeling Brain. London, Karnac, 2015

Tuckett D: Does anything go? Towards a framework for the more transparent assessment of psychoanalytic competence. Int J Psychoanal 86:31–49, 2005

Volkan V: Blind Trust. Charlottesville, VA, Pitchstone, 2004

Wallerstein RS: Psychoanalytic therapy research: a commentary. Contemporary Psychoanalysis 50(1–2):259–269, 2014

Weigert E: The goal of creativity in psychotherapy. Am J Psychoanal 24:4–14, 2014

Yeomans FE, Clarkin JF, Kernberg OF: Transference Focused Psychotherapy for Borderline Personality Disorder: A Clinical Guide. Washington, DC, American Psychiatric Publishing, 2015

Zagermann P (ed): The Future of Psychoanalysis: The Debate About the Training Analysis System. London, Karnac, 2017

Index

Page numbers printed in **boldface** type refer to tables or figures.

Acting out
    countertransference and intensity
        of, 74
    narcissistic personality disorder
        and, 178, 179
    transference analysis and, 12, 41
Affective dominance
    supervision and, 116–117
    TFP and interpretation of, 40,
        95–106
    transference analysis and, 11
Affect systems, and neurobiology,
    4–5, 16–18
Aggression
    Freud's concept of death drive
        and, 4, 21
    group psychology and, 225
    love relationships of narcissistic
        patients and, 173, 182
    "negative" affect systems and,
        16–17
    schizoid personality disorder
        and, 140
    supervision and, 120
    symbiotic transference and, 87
    transference analysis and, 9–10
Albright, Madeline, 227, 230
"Alternative DSM-5 Model for Per-
    sonality Disorders" (American
    Psychiatric Association 2013),
    64
Amygdala, and schizophrenia, 151
Anorexia nervosa, 154
Anthony, E.J., 194, 197

Antisocial personality disorder
    group psychology and, 210, 225,
        226–227
    syndrome of perversity in narcis-
        sistic patients and, 182
Applebaum, Ann and Steve, 195
Assessment, of reality testing, 147–
    148. See also Diagnosis; Evalua-
    tion
Austen Riggs Psychiatric Clinic
    (Massachusetts), 200

Bao-Lord, B., 225
Barchas, Jack, 201
Barranger, M. and W., 105
"Basic assumption groups," 215–217
Bauer, Steven, 200, 201
Behavior. See also Acting out; Aggres-
    sion
    inappropriate or problematic in
        love relationships, 174
    malignant narcissism and antiso-
        cial, 223, 225, 226–227
    transference analysis and pat-
        terns of, 9–14
"Benign delusional syndromes," and
    schizophrenia, 153
Bion, Wilfred, 95, 96, 100, 118, 194,
    197, 202, 207, 208, 215–217, 219
Blackmail, and love relationships,
    173–174
Body dysmorphic syndrome, 154
Bollas, C., 26

Bonding, and sexual relations, 174
Borderline personality disorder. *See
also* Borderline personality organization
  case example of, 73–75, 159–161
  eye contact in Zoom sessions, 102
  love relationships and, 171–172
  narcissism and, 76, 223
  MBT for, 110–111
  role reversals and interpretation
    of, 40
Borderline personality organization
  (BPO). *See also* Borderline personality disorder
  development of integrated self
    and, 66
  dyadic relationship and, 109–110
  dynamic unconscious and, 25, 29
  inpatient psychotherapeutic
    treatment and, 203
  outcome of psychoanalysis or
    TFP, **150**
  structural aspects of transference
    in, 72–75, 85–86
  supervision and, 121, 123, 127
Bosnia, and group psychology, 229
Boston Psychopathic Hospital, 192
Boundaries, and love relations, 170,
  174–175
Britton, R., 86
Bureaucracy, and group psychology,
  228
"Burnout" syndrome, and hospital
  staff, 198
Busch, Fred, 43, 247

Caligor, Eve, 36, 58, 248
Canetti, E., 222–223
Caretaker, love relationships and role
  of, 172
Carr, Arthur, 200
Case examples
  of borderline personality disor-
    der, 73–75, 159–161
  of narcissistic personality disor-
    der, 78–79, 87–88, 139, 161–
    162, 182–187

of neurotic personality structure,
  70–72
of paranoid schizophrenia, 89–90,
  154–156
of psychotic personality disorder,
  154–162
of schizoid personality disorder,
  83–85, 136–142, 143, 144
Castle Hospital (London), 193
Chavez, Hugo, 230
Chestnut Lodge Clinic, 192
Child and adolescent psychoanalysis,
  248–249
Children, and boundaries of love relationships, 174–175
Chinese Cultural Revolution, 225
Clarkin, John, 201
Cognitive-behavioral therapy, 199
Columbia University, 200
Community-based psychiatry movement, 199
Community meetings, and inpatient
  treatment, 196, 208
Community relations, and psychoan-
  alytic centers, 244
Competence, of psychoanalysts
  definition of professional, 234,
    235, 236
  evaluation of, 246–247
  standards for certification, 244–245
Conflicts, and love relationships of
  narcissistic patients, 170–171,
  179. *See also* Organizational
  structure and conflict
Containment, and basic techniques of
  psychoanalysis, 37
Cornell University. *See* Personality
  Disorders Institute
Countertransference
  borderline personality disorder
    and intensity of, 74
  difference of utilization in stan-
    dard psychoanalysis versus
    TFP, 44–45
  fundamental technical instru-
    ments of psychoanalysis and,
    36–37, 63

schizoid personality disorder
and, 82, 84–85, 144, 145
supervision and, 115, 119
training in standard psychoanalysis and TFP, 56–57
transference analysis and, 10–11
Couples therapy, 171
Creativity, and study of unconscious,
241–242
Crowds, and mass psychology, 214
Culture, influence of psychoanalysis
on, 233–234. *See also* Social systems

Dead mother syndrome, and dismantling of transference, 90–91
Defenses, object relations theory and
systematic interpretation of, 65,
66
Dependency, and Bion's theory of basic assumption groups, 216–217
Depression. *See* Major depression
with psychosis; Psychotic depression
Development
of affective memory accumulation, 7
of dynamic unconscious, 24–25
Diagnosis. *See also* Assessment; Initial
evaluation
psychotic personality organization and, 163–164
supervision and, 118
training in TFP and, 46–47
Dialectic behavior therapy, 199–200
Dishonesty, and leadership of mass
movements, 225–227
Dream analysis, 45, 97
Drives, and drive theory
Freud's theory of, 4, 20–21, 65
modification of classical motivational psychoanalytic theory
and, 4–5
Drug-induced psychosis, 154
DSM-5, and schizoid personality disorder, 134
Dulz, B., 204

Dyadic relationship, and TFP, 106–112
Dynamic psychotherapy for higher
personality pathology (DPHP),
69
Dynamic unconscious, 5, 22–29

Education, and research, 242–243. *See*
Psychoeducation; Training
Ego, superego, and id, concepts of in
object relations theory, 6, 8, 27, 66
Ego-syntonic aggression, and malig-
nant narcissism, 223
Empathy, and supervision, 126–127
Envy, and love relations of narcissistic
patients, 175–176, 178, 179, 182
Evaluation, of professional compe-
tence, 246–247. *See also* Initial
evaluation
"Expressive" psychotherapy, 63
Expressive-supportive psychother-
apy (Ex-SupP), **69**
Ezriel, H., 194, 197, 202, 207, 208

Fairbairn, W., 80, 81, 134, 142, 193
Fantasy
narcissistic sexual pathology and,
176
schizoid personality disorder
and, 135, 144, 145
Fenichel, Otto, 96
Fight-flight reactions, 17, 216
Foulkes, S.H., 194, 197
Free association
classical psychoanalytic technique and, 8
fundamental technical instruments
of psychoanalysis, 36–37
training in TFP and, 47–48
transference analysis and, 11, 13
Freud, Anna, 42
Freud, Sigmund, 4, 16, 20–21, 24, 65,
91, 95, 214–215, 219, 220–221,
238, 245

Gender identity, and love relationships, 166

Genetics, and schizophrenia, 151

Genocide, and group psychology, 228, 229

German depth psychology-oriented psychotherapy (TPOPSY), **69**

Germany
    group psychology and Nazi era, 227, 228, 229
    history of inpatient psychoanalytic treatment in, 191–192, 204–211
    psychoanalysts on faculty of universities in, 242

Grandiosity, and narcissistic personality disorder, 74–79, 146, 177, 178

Gratitude, and love relationships of narcissistic patients, 177

Great Britain, and inpatient psychoanalytic treatment of personality disorders, 192, 193

Green, André, 21, 53, 91

Group meetings, and inpatient treatment, 196, 197, 206

Group psychology
    dangers of to society, 227–231, 238
    development of theories of, 214–222
    leaders of and malignant narcissism, 222–227

Group psychotherapy, and TFP, 200, 202–203, 207–208

Group supervision
    importance of in learning process, 128–129, 247
    transference/countertransference issues and, 115

Guntrip, H., 80, 134, 142

Haran, Catherine, 200, 201

Hartocollis, Peter, 195

Harvard University. *See* Boston Psychopathic Hospital

Hippocampus, and neurobiology of affect system, 19, 22

Historical trauma, and group psychology, 226

Histrionic personality disorder, 98–99

Hitler, Adolf, 225, 227, 229, 230

Homeostatic mechanisms, and affect activation, 17

Horwitz, Leonard, 195

Hospital, analysis of as social system, 192–193, 206, 210. *See also* Inpatient treatment

Hunt, Howard, 200

Hypochondriasis, 154, 159

Id. *See* Ego

Idealization, and love relationships, 171, 172

Identity. *See also* Gender identity; Self
    group psychology and, 215, 218, 219–220, 221, 225
    psychoanalysts and professional, 248

Ideology, and group psychology, 219, 221–222, 226, 228, 229

Impulses, object relations theory and systematic interpretation of, 65

Infantile amnesia, 5, 24

Initial evaluation, and differences between standard psychotherapy and TFP, 38–39

Inpatient treatment, psychoanalytic approaches to for severe personality disorders, 191–211

Intensive psychotherapy, and psychotic transferences, 88–89

Internet, and group psychology, 228. *See also* Zoom

Interpretation
    affective dominance and, 95–106
    differences between standard psychoanalysis and TFP, 39–40
    fundamental technical instruments of psychoanalysis, 36–37
    schizoid personality disorder and, 82

ISIS (terrorist organization), 226

Jacobson, Edith, 51–52, 149, 151

Johnson, V.E., 166

Jones, Maxwell, 194, 198
Joseph, Betty, 41, 64, 144
Judicial system, and group psychology, 228

Kennedy, Lawrence, 195
Kernberg, Otto F., 62–63, 67, 195
Kernberg, Paulina, 195
Klein, Melanie, 7, 25, 28, 134, 135, 142, 148, 193–194, 200–201, 221
Kürner, J., 246

Language, personality disorders and systematic distortion of, 47–48. *See also* Verbal communication
Leaders, and leadership
    group psychology and, 215, 216–217, 218–220, 221, 222–231
    psychoanalytic centers and, 247–248
Libido
    Freud's description of affect systems and, 4
    "positive" affect systems and, 16–17
    transference analysis and, 9–10
Loewald, Hans, 39, 100
Love relationships. *See also* Social relationships
    narcissistic personalities and, 167–187
    technical neutrality and training in TFP, 55–56

Main, Thomas F., 193, 194, 195
Major depression with psychosis, 151, 154
Malignant narcissism. *See also* Narcissistic personality disorder
    leadership of mass movements and, 222–231
    love relationships and, 173
Managed care, impact of on psychiatric care, 199, 201
Manic syndrome, 154
Marx, Karl, 222

Mass movements, and Freud's theory of group psychology, 214–215
Masters, W.H., 166
McWilliams, N., 134
Memory. *See also* Working memory
    dynamic unconscious and, 22–23
    object relations theory and development of affective, 7
Menninger, Roy, 195
Menninger Clinic, 192, 195, 198
Menninger study, 63
Mentalization, and dyadic relationship in TFP, 106–112
Mentalization-based therapy (MBT)
    borderline personality disorganization and, 110–111
    dominant techniques of, **69**
    transference interpretation in TFP and, 50–51
Mental status interview, and reality testing, 147
Michels, Robert, 200
Microanalysis, and grandiose self in narcissistic personality disorder, 78
Moscovici, S., 222, 238
Multi-culturalism, and group psychology, 230

Narcissistic personality disorder. *See also* Malignant narcissism; Negative narcissism
    affective dominance and, 97
    case examples of, 78–79, 87–88, 139, 161–162, 182–187
    grandiosity and, 74–79, 146, 177, 178
    leadership and group psychology, 223
    love relationships and sexual relations, 167–187
    modifications in psychoanalytic technique for, 29
    transference analysis and, 12, 13
    transference structures and, 75–79, 87–88
Negative narcissism, and Freud's concept of death drive, 21

Neurobiology
  affect systems and, 4–5, 16–18
  dynamic unconscious and, 22–29
  representation of self and others, 18–20
  revisions of psychoanalytic theory and, 29–30, 237–238
  schizophrenia and, 151–153
Neurotic personality organization
  affective dominance and, 96–98
  case example of classic psychoanalytic treatment for, 70–72
  internalized object relationships and, 110
  outcome of psychoanalysis or TFP, **150**
  supervision and, 120, 122–123
Neurotransmitters, and schizophrenia, 152–153
New York State Psychiatric Institute, 200
Novotnik, Peter, 195
Nursing staff, and inpatient treatment of personality disorders, 208–209, 210

Object relations theory
  basic psychoanalytic concepts of drive derivatives and defensive impulses, 65
  concept of self and, 6, 8, 18–20
  defense mechanisms of BPO, 66
  overview of theory and technique of TFP, 3–8
  reality testing and, 148
  transference analysis in TFP and, 8–14
Obsessive-compulsive personality disorder, 127
Ogden, T.H., 28
Organizational structure and conflict, as specialization, 249

Panksepp, J., 24
"Parallel process," and supervision, 118, 121

Paranoid personality disorder, 13, 222, 223
Paranoid psychosis, 154, 157
Paranoid-schizoid position
  group psychology and, 221
  Klein's description of, 7, 66, 135, 142, 221
  schizoid personality disorder and, 134, 135–136, 141, 142, 144, 146
Paranoid schizophrenia
  case examples of, 89–90, 154–156
  intensive psychotherapy for, 89–90
Paranoid transference, and narcissistic patients, 179–180
Personality disorders. *See also* Antisocial personality disorder; Borderline personality disorder; Histrionic personality disorder; Narcissistic personality disorder; Obsessive-compulsive personality disorder; Paranoid personality disorder; Psychoanalysis and psychoanalytic theory; Psychotic personality disorder; Schizoid personality disorder
  advantages of TFP in initial evaluation of, 39
  affective dominance and, 98, 99, 102
  countertransference reactions and, 44–45
  psychoanalytic approaches to inpatient treatment of, 191–211
  supervision in severe cases of, 122
  systematic distortion of language in, 47–48
  transference analysis and, 10, 42
Personality Disorders Institute (Cornell University), 64, 144, 160, 166, 201
Perversity, syndrome of, 182
Power
  love relationships and, 172–173
  mass movements and, 215, 227

Prefrontal cortex, and neurobiology, 19, 23, 24, 151–152
Professional development, and psychoanalytic centers, 244
Projective identification, and inpatient treatment, 196
Psychoanalysis and psychoanalytic theory. *See also* Countertransference; Interpretation; Object relations theory; Personality disorders; Technical neutrality; Training; Transference analysis; Transference-focused psychotherapy (TFP); Transference structures
countertransference utilization and, 44–45
current crisis in, 233–236
development as psychoanalyst and, 127
differences between standard and TFP, 36–45, 57–58
dynamic unconscious and, 22–24
Freud's theory of death drive, 20–21
group psychology and, 214–222
implications of transference structures for, 62–68
inpatient treatment of severe personality disorders and, 191–211
modified approaches to, 236–237
neurobiology and, 16–18, 29–30, 237–238
potential solutions to theoretical challenges, 237–249
representation of self and others, 18–20
specialization within treatment approaches, 113–114
use of term "standard," 36, 62–63, 64, 91–92
Psychoanalytic centers, and research, 243–244, 247–248. *See also* Menninger Clinic; New York Psychiatric Institute; Personality Disorders Institute

Psychodynamic psychotherapy, 121–122, 142–144
Psychoeducation, and inpatient treatment, 210
Psychopathic transferences, 13
Psychopharmacology, for psychosis and schizophrenia, 152–153, 199
Psychosis. *See also* Psychotic personality disorder; Psychotic personality organization; Psychotic transferences; Schizophrenia
development of psychopharmacology for, 199
use of term, 147
Psychosocial environment, and affect systems, 18
Psychotic depression, 151, 154
Psychotic functioning, use of term, 147
Psychotic personality disorder, 153, 154–162
Psychotic personality organization
case examples of, 162, 163–164
outcome of psychoanalysis or TFP, **150**
reality testing and, 151, 153–154
Psychotic transferences
case examples of psychotic personality disorder and, 154, 158, 159, 161, 162–163
transference structure and, 88–90, 157
use of term, 85, **87**

Reality testing
assessment of, 147–148
differentiated from relationship to reality, 148
psychotic personality disorder and, 147, 153–154, 163
representation of self and, 149, 151
transference analysis and, 41–42
Regression
leadership of large groups and, 224–227
transference analysis and, 12–13

Relational psychoanalytic approach, and interpretation of counter-transference, 64

Religion, and psychotic personality disorder, 153

Repetition compulsion, and supervision, 117

Research, and development of psychoanalytic theories and techniques, 241, 242–244

Resistance, and classification of basic techniques of psychoanalysis, 37

Rey, J.H., 80

Rice, A. Kenneth, 195

Rioch, Margaret J., 195

Role reversals
borderline personality disorder and interpretation of, 40
dyadic relationship and, 108, 109
love relationships and, 172–173

Rosenfeld, Herbert, 89, 151, 192

Roth, Gerhard, 29

Rwanda, and group psychology, 229

Schizoid personality disorder
affective dominance and, 101
case examples of, 83–85, 136–142, 143, 144
descriptive characteristics of, 133–136
dynamic unconscious and, 26
modifications in psychoanalytic technique for, 29
psychodynamic considerations in treatment of, 142–144
transference structures and, 79–85
TFP for treatment of, 144–146

Schizophrenia. *See also* Paranoid schizophrenia
case examples of psychotic personality disorder and, 156–158
dynamic unconscious and, 26
intensive psychotherapy for, 89
neurobiology and, 151–153
outcome of psychoanalysis or TFP for, **150**, 153

paranoid-schizoid mechanisms and defensive operations of, 148

Schwartz, M., 192–193

Searles, Harold, 88–89, 90, 157, 158

"SEEKING" system, 17

"Selected fact," affective dominance and concept of, 96

Self
borderline transference and, **73**
development of integrated, 66
dynamic unconscious and, 23–24, 27
narcissistic personality disorder and grandiose, 74–79, 177
neurobiology of affect systems and, 18
neurotic transference and, **71**
object relations theory and concept of, 6, 8, 18–20
psychotic transference and, **87**
reality testing and, 149, 151
schizoid personality disorder and, 80, **81**
symbiotic transference and, 85, **86**

Self-representation, and transference analysis, 40–41

Semelin, Jacques, 227, 229, 230–231

Seminars, on psychoanalytic and psychotherapeutic technique, 129

Separation-panic, and negative affect systems, 17

September 11, 2001 terrorist attack, 219

Sexual life. *See* Love relationships

Silence, and affective dominance, 103–104

Skills training, and inpatient treatment, 210

Snyder, Timothy, 227, 231

Social organizations, malignant narcissism and leadership of, 224, 230

Social media, and group psychology, 228

Social relationships, and schizoid personality disorder, 80, 83, 134–135, 144. *See also* Love relationships

Social systems. *See also* Culture
　group psychology and, 219, 221,
　　227, 238
　hospital as, 192–193, 206, 210
Social workers, role of in inpatient
　treatment, 209
Sociology, and psychoanalytic theory,
　238–239
Solms, Mark, 24
Somatization, and transference anal-
　ysis, 12
Soviet Union, and group psychology,
　228
Spillius, Elizabeth, 153
Stalin, Joseph, 225, 229
"Standard" psychoanalysis, use of
　term, 36, 62–63, 64, 91–92
Standards for certification, 244–245
Stanton, A.M., 192–193
Stone, Michael, 89, 153, 200–201
Sullivan, Harry, 192
Superego. *See* Ego
Supervision. *See also* Training
　different approaches to psychoan-
　　alytic treatment and, 113–117
　frequent problems in, 117–126
　limitations of, 126–129
　role of in psychoanalytic educa-
　　tion, 247
Supportive psychotherapy (SPY), 68,
　69
Sutherland, J.D., 194, 195, 197, 202
Symbiotic transferences, 13, 85–88
Symbols, and "protosymbols" of
　mass movements, 220

Task groups, and inpatient treatment,
　196
Tavistock Clinic (London), 194–195
Technical neutrality
　differences between standard psy-
　　choanalysis and TFP, 42–43
　fundamental technical instru-
　　ments of psychoanalysis and,
　　36–37, 63
　group psychotherapy and, 203

schizoid personality disorder
　and, 145
supervision and, 122
training in TFP and, 54–56
transference analysis and, 11, 12
TFP. *See* Transference-focused psy-
　chotherapy
Therapeutic alliance, and basic tech-
　niques of psychoanalysis, 37. *See
　also* Therapeutic relationship
Therapeutic community, and tradi-
　tional medical model, 198
Therapeutic frame, and transference
　analysis, 11
Therapeutic relationship. *See also*
　Therapeutic alliance
　assumption of normal as precon-
　　dition for TFP, 100
　supervision and, 119
Ticho, Ernst and Gertrude, 195
Totalitarian systems, and group psy-
　chology, 228
Total object relationship, and BPO, 73
Total transference, TFP and concept
　of analysis of, 41, 55
Training, of psychoanalytic therapists.
　See also Supervision
　definition of professional compe-
　　tence and, 234, 235, 236
　differences between standard psy-
　　choanalysis and TFP, 45–57
　evaluation of competence, 246–247
　inclusion of modified approaches
　　in, 236–237
　new curriculum proposed for,
　　245–246
　recent changes in, 234–236
　requirement for personal psycho-
　　analysis, 247
　specialization and, 248–249
Transference analysis. *See also* Psy-
　chopathic transferences; Psy-
　chotic transferences; Symbiotic
　transferences; Total transference;
　Transference structures
　differences between standard psy-
　　choanalysis and TFP, 40–42

Transference analysis *(continued)*
  fundamental technical instruments of psychoanalysis and, 36–37, 63
  psychosis induced in course of, 154
  representation of self and others, 20
  schizoid personality disorder and, 145, 146
  supervision and, 115
  theoretical approach of TFP and, 8–14
  training in TFP and, 52–54
Transference-focused psychotherapy (TFP)
  affective dominance and, 40, 95–106
  basic psychoanalytic techniques and, 240
  BPO and, 29, 73, 75, **150**
  countertransference utilization and, 44–45
  differences between standard psychoanalysis and, 36–44, 57–58
  dominant techniques of compared to other methodologies, **69**
  dyadic relationship and mentalization, 106–112
  group therapy and, 202–203
  Menninger study and development of, 63
  neurotic personality organization and, **150**
  overview of theory and techniques of, 3–8
  Personality Disorders Institute and development of, 201
  psychotic personality organization and, **150**
  schizoid personality disorder and, 144–146
  schizophrenia and, **150**
  training issues and, 45–57
  transference analysis and, 8–14
Transference psychosis. *See* Psychotic transference
Transference structures. *See also* Transference analysis

application of psychoanalytic techniques and, 62–68
  BPO and, 72–75
  dead mother syndrome and dismantling of, 90–91
  narcissistic personality disorder and, 75–79
  neurotic personality organization and, 70–72
  schizoid personality disorder and, 79–85
  symbiotic transferences and, 85–88
Traumatization, unconscious conflicts and early experiences of, 7, 24, 25, 26, 28, 52
Trust, and love relations, 170
Tuckett, David, 41, 246
Turquet, Pierre, 217–219, 221, 227

Unconscious intrapsychic conflict, revision of classical theory of, 4–5. *See also* Dynamic unconscious
United Nations, 231
"Us" versus "them," and group psychology, 216, 220

Value systems, and technical neutrality, 55
Verbal communication, and advantages of standard psychoanalytic training for TFP therapist, 47–48. *See also* Language
Volkan, Vamik, 219–221, 238

Wallerstein, R., 63
Working memory. *See also* Memory
  affect systems and function of, 18
  dynamic unconscious and, 23

Yale Psychiatric Hospital, 193
Yeomans, Frank, 201
Yugoslavia, and group psychology, 229

Zoom, and psychoanalytic treatment, 101–102